Band 29, Heft 2, April 2013

Viszeralmedizin

Gastrointestinal Medicine and Surgery

Schwerpunkt

J. Ricke, Magdeburg
N.P. Malek, Tübingen
U.P. Neumann, Aachen
(Hrsg.)

Hepatozelluläres Karzinom – ein interdisziplinäres Krankheitsbild

Eingeladene Beiträge

Interdisziplinäres Gespräch

Weitere Rubriken

Fallbericht

Originalarbeit

News/Ticker

Tagungen und Kongresse

KARGER

Basel · Freiburg · Paris · London · New York · New Delhi · Bangkok · Beijing · Tokyo · Kuala Lumpur · Singapore · Sydney

Band 29, Heft 2, April 2013

Viszeralmedizin

Gastrointestinal Medicine and Surgery

Gegründet 1984 als «Chirurgische Gastroenterologie mit interdisziplinären Gesprächen» durch A. Akovbiantz, H. Denk, K.-J. Paquet und C.E. Zöckler

S. Karger GmbH
Postfach, 79095 Freiburg

Editorial Office
Alexander Eitner
a.eitner@karger.com

KARGER

Basel · Freiburg · Paris · London · New York · New Delhi · Bangkok · Beijing · Tokyo · Kuala Lumpur · Singapore · Sydney

Transforming Vesalius

The medical revolution of the 16th century brought to life for the 21st century

500 YEARS Vesalius

KARGER
Medical & Scientific Publishers

ANDREAS VESALIUS

The Fabric of the Human Body

An Annotated Translation of the 1543 and 1555 Editions with Vesalius' Own Notes for a Never Published Third Edition

DANIEL H. GARRISON
MALCOLM H. HAST

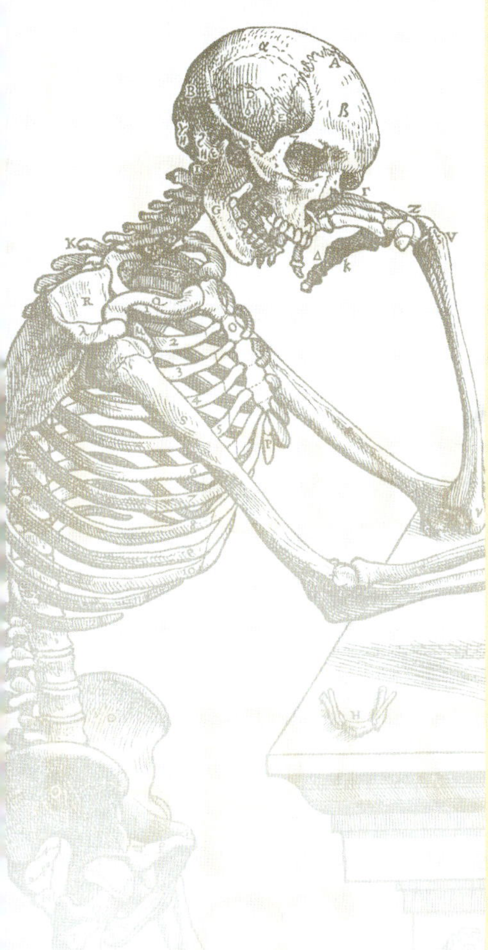

The Fabric of the Human Body, an annotated translation of Andreas Vesalius' *De humani corporis fabrica*, will be published by Karger Publishers in autumn 2013. The new book recreates the masterpiece of science and art for the first time in a way that is understandable to 21st century readers who do not have any knowledge of Latin.

The texts of both the 1543 and the 1555 editions have been translated with the utmost care by Northwestern University Professors Emeritus Daniel H. Garrison and Malcolm H. Hast, a task they completed in over 20 years of painstaking and dedicated work.

Annotations give the reader keen insight into just how innovative *De humani corporis fabrica* was, and high-resolution digital scans of the almost 300 woodcuts provide the images with a sharpness they never had before.

- First English translation of the 1543 and 1555 editions with detailed annotations and added notes for a never published third edition – all in one publication
- Different colors allow easy identification of notes specifically relevant to the 1543 and 1555 editions
- A modern design and high-resolution digital scans make *The Fabric of the Human Body* accessible to every scholar, library, and book lover
- *Nomina Anatomica* and *Terminologia Anatomica* are included for the first time, clearly providing Vesalius' description with the appropriate modern medical terminology
- With prefaces by the translators and extensive introductions by medical historians Vivian Nutton and Nancy Siraisi

Vesalius, A.
The Fabric of the Human Body
An Annotated Translation of the 1543 and 1555 Editions of "De Humani Corporis Fabrica", by D. H. Garrison and M. H. Hast

Approx. 1,400 pages in two books
Hard cover with slip case
12 × 17" / 315 × 435 mm
Approx. 30 lbs / 14 kg

List price: CHF 1,500.– / EUR 1,250.– / USD 1,650.00
Pre-publication price: CHF 1,125.– / EUR 935.– / USD 1,235.00
Valid until end of September 2013
Postage and handling included
VAT & import taxes excluded
EUR price for Germany,
USD price for USA only
ISBN 978-3-318-02246-9

www.karger.com

www.vesalius-fabrica.com

- For more information on *The Fabric of the Human Body*, Vesalius, and the 16th century
- For easy ordering with a special pre-publication price
- For the Library Recommendation

KI 12302_SKD

Viszeralmedizin
Gastrointestinal Medicine and Surgery

Inhalt · Contents

Band 29, Heft 2, April 2013

Schwerpunkt: Hepatozelluläres Karzinom – ein interdisziplinäres Krankheitsbild

Herausgeber: Ricke, J. (Magdeburg); Malek, N.P. (Tübingen); Neumann, U.P. (Aachen)

Vol. 29, Issue 2, April 2013

Focus: Hepatocellular Carcinoma – an Interdisciplinary Disease Pattern

Editors: Ricke, J. (Magdeburg); Malek, N.P. (Tübingen); Neumann, U.P. (Aachen)

KARGER
Fax +49 761 4 52 07 14
Information@Karger.com
www.karger.com

Accessible online at:
www.karger.com/vim

Viszeralmedizin
Gastrointestinal Medicine and Surgery

Inhalt · Contents

Band 29, Heft 2, April 2013

Vol. 29, Issue 2, April 2013

KARGER
Fax +49 761 4 52 07 14
Information@Karger.com
www.karger.com

Accessible online at:
www.karger.com/vim

Viszeralmedizin
Gastrointestinal Medicine and Surgery

Editorial

Viszeralmedizin 2013;29:71
DOI: 10.1159/000350809

Online publiziert: 3. April 2013

Hepatozelluläres Karzinom – ein interdisziplinäres Krankheitsbild

Jens Ricke[a] Nisar Peter Malek[b] Ulf Peter Neumann[c]

[a] Klinik für Radiologie und Nuklearmedizin, Universitätsklinikum Magdeburg AöR,
[b] Abteilung Innere Medizin 1, Medizinische Universitätsklinik, Tübingen,
[c] Klinik für Allgemein-, Viszeral- und Transplantationschirurgie, Universitätsklinikum Aachen, Deutschland

Das hepatozelluläre Karzinom (HCC) ist für Ärzte und Wissenschaftler eine große Herausforderung, da es wie kein zweiter Tumor eine außerordentlich enge Verzahnung der Disziplinen erfordert. In den letzten Jahren hat es erhebliche Erkenntnisfortschritte in der Pathogenese, Diagnostik und interdisziplinären Therapie gegeben. Aufgrund der in der Regel vorliegenden Koinzidenz der Krankheitsbilder in der Kombination eines aggressiven Tumorleidens auf dem Boden einer meist schwierig zu beherrschenden Lebererkrankung besteht eine besondere Herausforderung nicht nur in fachlicher und intellektueller, sondern insbesondere auch in logistischer Hinsicht.

Wie viele Kliniken leisten sich heute echte interdisziplinäre Konzepte mit kombinierten Ambulanzen und Stationen, um tatsächlich zu garantieren, dass Patienten von den Spezialisten der unterschiedlichen beteiligten Fächer gesehen werden? Im vorliegenden Heft hoffen wir deutlich zu machen, dass insbesondere in dieser interdisziplinären Zusammenarbeit nicht nur der Schlüssel zum Verständnis der Erkrankung, sondern auch zu einer besseren Therapie liegt.

Welches Krankheitsbild zeichnet sich schon durch den traurigen Ruhm aus, gegebenenfalls eine breite Anforderungskette von den Grundlagen der Virusprävention und -behandlung über die molekularen Tiefen der Karzinogenese und Angiogenese bis hin zu komplexesten Infrastrukturleistungen wie die Versorgung der Patienten vor, während und nach einer Lebertransplantation zu erfordern?

Das vorliegende Heft kann all diese Herausforderungen naturgemäß nicht erschöpfend diskutieren. Wir freuen uns aber, Ihnen eine Fülle von Anregungen nicht nur für die Versorgung der Ihnen anvertrauten Patienten, sondern auch für die Weiterentwicklung der diagnostischen und therapeutischen Möglichkeiten bei HCCs mitgeben zu können.

KARGER
Fax +49 761 4 52 07 14
Information@Karger.com
www.karger.com

1662-6664/13/0292-0071$38.00/0

Accessible online at:
www.karger.com/vim

Prof. Dr. med. Jens Ricke
Klinik für Radiologie und Nuklearmedizin
Universitätsklinikum Magdeburg AöR
Leipziger Straße 44, 39120 Magdeburg, Deutschland
jens.ricke@med.ovgu.de

Viszeralmedizin
Gastrointestinal Medicine and Surgery

Review Article · Übersichtsarbeit

Viszeralmedizin 2013;29:72–77
DOI: 10.1159/000350830

Online publiziert: 15. April 2013

Imaging in Hepatocellular Carcinoma: Guidelines and Future Prospects

Carlo Bartolozzi   Valentina Battaglia

Diagnostic and Interventional Radiology, University of Pisa, Italy

Keywords
Liver · Cirrhosis · Diagnosis ·
Hepatocellular carcinoma, HCC · Magnetic resonance, MR

Summary
Background: Non-invasive diagnosis of hepatocellular carcinoma (HCC) in cirrhosis is nowadays the option of choice, as reported by both Western and Eastern guidelines. **Methods:** Currently, the diagnosis is still focused on the detection of the typical, neoplastic, vascular pattern, characterized by lesion hypervascularization in the arterial phase and by wash-out in the late vascular phase, by means of multidetector computed tomography (MDCT) or magnetic resonance (MR) imaging. In cases of atypical nodules, Western international guidelines suggest, depending on the cases, to perform a second imaging examination, but not contrast-enhanced ultrasound (CEUS), or biopsy tissue sampling. On the contrary, Eastern guidelines have additionally included RES(reticuloendothelial system)-targeted ultrasound or MR examination or hepatobiliary MR imaging for these difficult cases. **Results:** On the basis of new findings regarding the histological changes occurring in the pathway towards nodular malignancy, new hepatospecific contrast agents are routinely applied in MR studies, allowing to explore cellular metabolic function also in atypical hypoperfused nodules. **Conclusions:** In the near future, hepatobiliary MR imaging with hepatocyte-selective contrast agents might be considered the best choice to classify preneoplastic, low-risk lesions or atypical nodules with a high potential of malignancy.

Schlüsselwörter
Leber · Zirrhose · Diagnose ·
Hepatozelluläres Karzinom, HCC · Magnetresonanz, MR

Zusammenfassung
Hintergrund: Die nichtinvasive Diagnose des hepatozellulären Karzinoms (HCC) in Zirrhose stellt heutzutage die erste Behandlung der Wahl dar, wie sowohl in westlichen als auch in östlichen Leitlinien berichtet wird. **Methoden:** Derzeit fokussiert sich die Diagnose mittels Multidetektor-Computertomographie (MDCT) oder Magnetresonanztomographie (MRT) nach wie vor auf die Detektion des typischen, neoplastischen, vaskulären Musters, das durch Hypervaskularisation von Läsionen in der arteriellen Phase und durch «wash-out» in der späten vaskulären Phase gekennzeichnet ist. Bei atypischen Knoten schlagen die westlichen internationalen Leitlinien je nach Fall eine zweite bildgebende Untersuchung ohne kontrastverstärkten Ultraschall (CEUS) oder eine Stanzbiopsie vor. Im Gegensatz hierzu haben die östlichen Leitlinien RES(retikuloendotheliales System)-spezifisches Ulltraschall- oder MR-Kontrastmittel oder die hepatobiliäre MRT aufgenommen. **Ergebnisse:** Auf der Grundlage der neuen Erkenntnisse bezüglich der histologischen Veränderungen, die im Verlauf der Entstehung von malignen Knötchen auftreten, werden neue hepatospezifische Kontrastmittel routinemäßig in MRT-Studien angewandt; dies erlaubt die Erforschung der zellulären metabolischen Funktion auch in atypischen Knoten. **Schlussfolgerungen:** In der nahen Zukunft könnte sich die hepatobiliäre MRT mit Hepatozyten-spezifischen Kontrastmitteln als Methode der Wahl für präneoplastische Läsionen mit niedrigem Risiko und atypische Knoten mit hohem Risiko für Malignität etablieren.

KARGER
Fax +49 761 4 52 07 14
Information@Karger.com
www.karger.com

1662-6664/13/0292-0072$38.00/0

Accessible online at:
www.karger.com/vim

Prof. Carlo Bartolozzi, MD
Diagnostic and Interventional Radiology, University of Pisa
Via Paradisa 2, 56100 Pisa, Italy
carlo.bartolozzi@med.unipi.it

Introduction

Hepatocellular carcinoma (HCC) is one of the most common malignant neoplasms worldwide, with an estimated incidence of more than 500,000 new cases per year.

The most common background in which the neoplasm arises is represented by cirrhosis. In Western countries cirrhosis is mainly due to chronic infection caused by hepatitis C virus (HCV), followed by chronic hepatitis B virus (HBV) infection and alcohol abuse; other causes of chronic liver injury frequently related to the development of HCC are represented by cholestatic, autoimmune, and metabolic disorders as well as nonalcoholic steatohepatitis (NASH) [1, 2].

Clinically, HCC does not show a specific presentation as the symptoms of the underlying cirrhosis are frequently dominant. As a consequence, scheduled surveillance of selected patients is currently the major practical approach for an early diagnosis of a neoplasm, as suggested in all of the international guidelines [3–5].

HCC Screening

Algorithms proposed by different guidelines, which might slightly differ in terms of target screening population as well as management of small detected nodules, have been employed to assist in the detection of small liver nodules found during surveillance.

The recently updated guidelines, issued by the American Association for the Study of Liver Diseases (AASLD), identify those affected by cirrhosis or by NASH as well as those affected by chronic HBV or HCV infection, even without an evidence of cirrhosis, as high-risk patients [4]. While a different surveillance management of HBV patients was suggested in the past, nowadays the time interval for surveillance reported by Western international guidelines, i.e. AASLD and EASL/EORTC (European Association for the Study of the Liver and European Organization for Research and Treatment of Cancer), is 4–6 months, independently of the cause of liver damage, since retrospective studies have demonstrated no benefit from a closer follow-up in terms of survival [3, 4, 6, 7].

On the contrary, Eastern guidelines, issued by the Asian Pacific Association for the Study of the Liver (APASL), indicate as appropriate an ultrasound (US) follow-up, performed every 3 months [5].

Selected patients do benefit from a prospective screening as it increases the possibility for early diagnosis of a neoplasm, allowing access to several, personalized, therapeutic options [8, 9].

In the past few years, both US examination and measurement of alpha-fetoprotein (AFP) levels were considered as the two main screening tools in the surveillance of cirrhotic patients.

Several studies have shown the limited role of AFP because of its poor specificity and low positive predictive value (PPV) in assessing the presence of a neoplasm specifically in a low-prevalence population such as in Western Europe; as a result, measurement of AFP has been removed from Western guidelines [10, 11].

Again, US, because of its low cost, its widely spread availability, and the absence of related risks, is considered as the unique and most appropriate approach for screening cirrhotic patients, showing otherwise a wide range of sensitivity (ranging between 58 and 89%), mainly related to the skills of the operator [12].

On the contrary, multidetector computed tomography (MDCT) and magnetic resonance (MR) imaging, despite their high reliability in diagnostic assessment, are not recommended as screening tools because of their sustained costs and possibly related harms such as radiation exposure and adverse events of contrast agents.

HCC Diagnosis

The development of a neoplasm in cirrhosis is a long-lasting process that might take months or even years. The continuous inflammatory stimulation which is caused by chronic HCV/HBV infections determines a chronic injury of hepatocytes and stromal liver cells. Many asynchronous cellular changes occur along the pathway from normal hepatocytes to neoplastic cells so that different types of hepatocellular nodules can be contemporarily present in a cirrhotic parenchyma: regenerative nodules, low-grade dysplastic nodules (LGDN), high-grade dysplastic nodules (HGDN), early HCC and, finally, overt HCC.

Particularly, HGDN nodules as well as early HCC are considered as premalignant and early malignant nodules since foci of HCC can be found inside HGDNs, while in cases of early HCC, usually all typical vascular changes have not yet occurred, unless the cells show signs of malignant degeneration [13, 14].

On the contrary, a decrease of portal venous supply in overt HCC (although still present only in very well differentiated lesions) and the development of neoangiogenesis, characterized by the presence of unpaired arteries and consistent arteriovenous shunts, is well established [14].

On the basis of such peculiar, microscopic, vascular architecture, non-invasive diagnosis of HCC in liver cirrhosis is actually demanded to perform post-contrastographic, dynamic imaging techniques, which are considered as the standard of reference.

Diagnostic MDCT should be performed by examining at least three phases (arterial, portal venous, and late phase) and by fixing the acquisition timing after contrast injection. Depending on the necessity to analyze arterial feeders as well as to obtain a vascular mapping of the liver, an early arterial phase should also be included in the protocol [15].

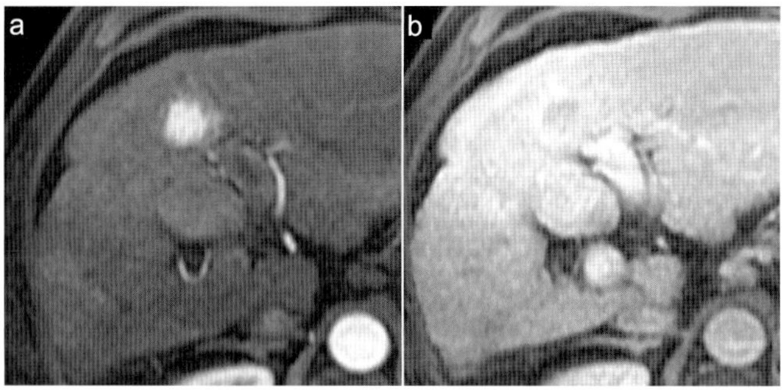

Fig. 1. Typical HCC enhancement pattern during dynamic MR study. Nodule within segment IV shows (**a**) a clear-cut enhancement on arterial phase and (**b**) a wash-out in the late vascular phase.

Similarly, in a standard post-contrastographic, dynamic MR study, performed with a high-field scanner (1.5T–3T), the same three vascular phases should be acquired. Due to the high temporal resolution of the system, a continuous acquisition after contrast agent injection is frequently carried out, independently of a fixed timing [16].

The so-called typical neoplastic pattern, characterized by a wash-in of early lesions in the arterial phase and a wash-out in the portal venous/late phases, has shown a PPV of 100% for a diagnosis of neoplasm, independently of the dimensions and grading of the lesions (fig. 1) [17, 18].

It should be noted that none of the guidelines reports which cross-sectional imaging modality between MDCT and MR should be applied in order to evaluate a suspected nodule detected during US surveillance; however, it is strongly recommended to perform both examinations in the case of lesions <2 cm by following dedicated acquisition protocols, possibly at specialized centers [4]. The EASL/EORTC guidelines recommend that only in centers of excellence with 'high-end radiological equipment' the assessment of nodules <2 cm should be performed with one imaging modality only [3, 4]. In case of doubt a biopsy must follow.

Dynamic MR and MDCT studies show a similar sensitivity in the detection of a typical, neoplastic, vascular pattern ranging between 44 and 62% as well as between 44 and 53%, respectively, although MR has been proven to be superior in assessing a correct diagnosis, especially in nodules smaller than 2 cm [19].

The latest EASL/EORTC as well as the AASLD guidelines have removed contrast-enhanced ultrasound (CEUS) from the diagnostic algorithm of HCC since it does not reliably differentiate between HCC and cholangiocellular carcinoma, showing identical wash-out phenomena; nevertheless, due to the high sensitivity of the technique in the detection of microcirculation, such a method can be suggested as a method of problem solving in suspected cases not showing hypervascularization in the arterial phase during MDCT or MR, especially in nodules smaller than 2 cm (fig. 2).

Moreover, CEUS evaluation, carried out during US examination, can be helpful in the differential diagnosis of other liver nodules that might be present in cirrhotic livers, such as hemangiomas, which are immediately characterized and ruled out from a subsequent, diagnostic work-up [20].

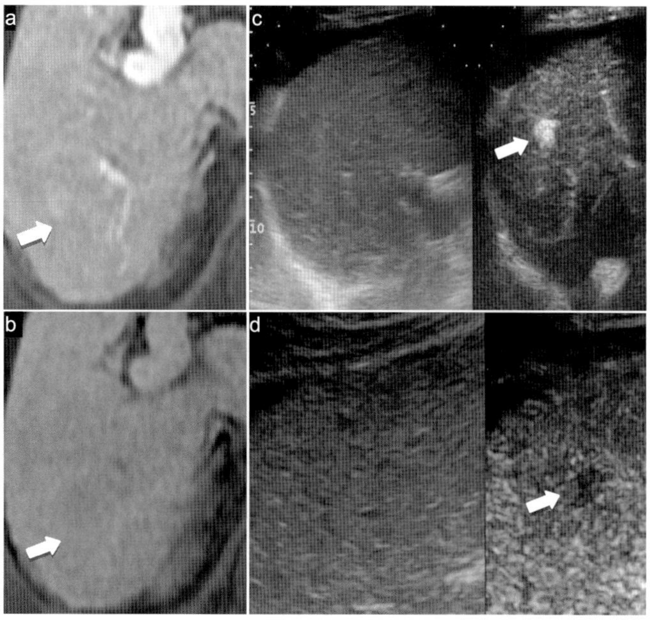

Fig. 2. Usefulness of CEUS. **a** At MR examination, a nodule (white arrow) in the arterial phase does not show a clear-cut enhancement. **b** In the late vascular phase, it shows as mildly hypointense. **c,d** However, at CEUS examination, performed 10 days after MR, the nodule is (**c**) typically hypervascular in the arterial phase and (**d**) hypoechoic in the late phase.

If the typical hallmarks of HCC at dynamic imaging are approved by all current guidelines, significant differences in the management of detected nodules at US surveillance on the basis of the dimensions of the nodules are appreciable among different diagnostic algorithms.

Regarding the EASL guidelines, the threshold of evaluating detected nodules by means of a single imaging technique is in fact 2 cm, while smaller nodules (between 1 and 2 cm) should be investigated by two imaging modalities. Nodules smaller than 1 cm should undergo a scheduled follow-up by US instead [3].

On the contrary, the AASLD guidelines suggest that the detection of the typical enhancement pattern at one single imaging modality in nodules larger than 1 cm can be considered as sufficient to formulate a diagnosis of neoplasm [4].

Finally, eastern guidelines disregard the dimensions of the nodules because the diagnosis of malignancy could be assessed even in lesions smaller than 1 cm in the case of a typical enhancement pattern during the dynamic imaging evaluation [5].

Since only two-thirds of HCCs are reported to show a typical pattern, the guidelines have furthermore focused on the attention concerning atypical nodules, which are hypovascular in the arterial phase, presenting again striking differences in management [2, 21].

While both EASL/EORTC and AASLD guidelines, focusing strongly on the dynamic pattern of the nodules, suggest biopsy as the third diagnostic step in the case of atypical nod-

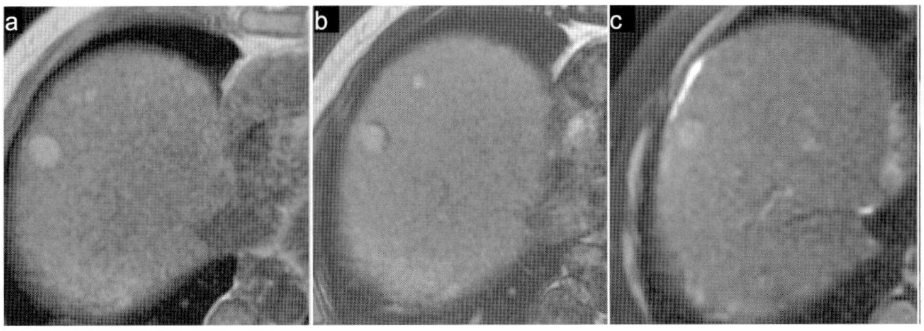

Fig. 3. Baseline MR examination. On baseline sequence, the small HCC nodule shows (**a**) as hyperintense on an in-phase T1-weighted image because of glycogen content, while on out-phase (**b**), the anterior part is hypointense due to the fat component within the lesion. Hyperintensity of the nodule on baseline T2-weighted image (**c**) is due to hypercellularity.

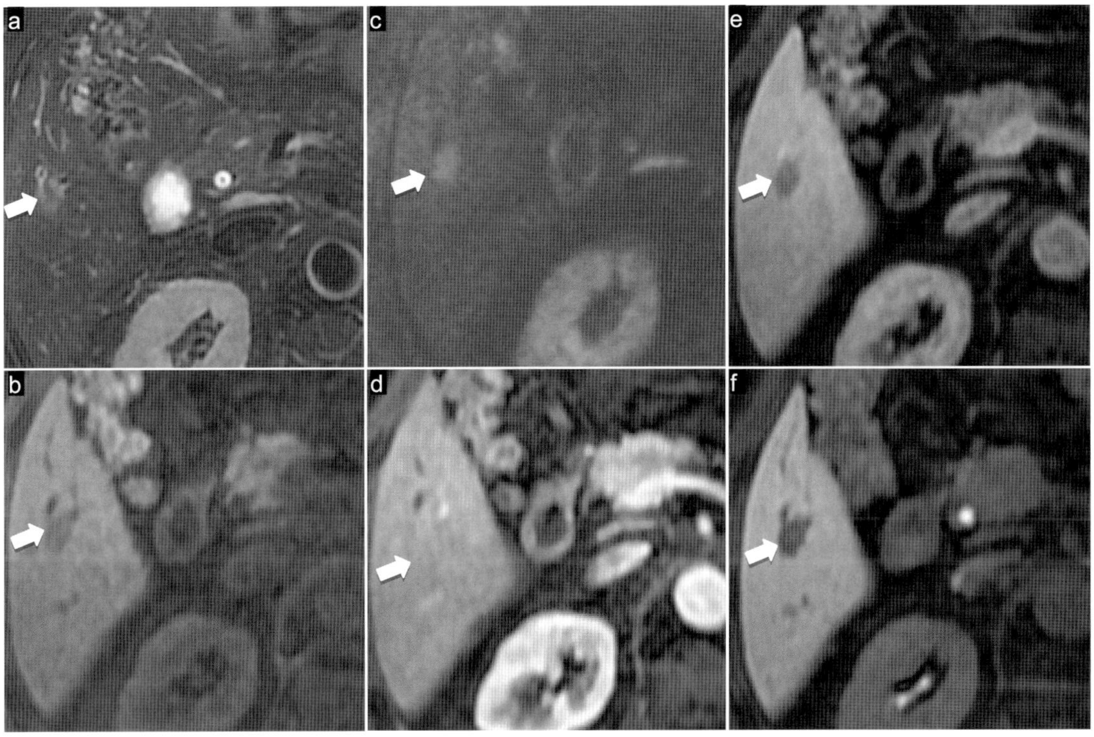

Fig. 4. Baseline and post-contrastographic examination of an atypical nodule within cirrhosis. The nodule (white arrow) shows (**a**) as hyperintense on baseline T2-weighted image, (**b**) as hypointense on baseline T1-weighted image, (**c**) a restriction of diffusivity at DWI (**b**, 800), and (**e**, **f**) as hypointense in the late dynamic and hepatobiliary phase. Despite all imaging findings fit in with a diagnosis of HCC, the lack of hypervascularization in the arterial phase (**d**) does not allow a diagnosis of neoplasm. Biopsy established a diagnosis of HGDN.

ules larger than 1 cm, the APASL and the Japanese guidelines have introduced new diagnostic tools.

Particularly, hypovascular nodules should be investigated regardless of size by applying RES- or hepatocyte-specific contrast agents during MR examinations or CEUS using Sonazoid [5].

Nevertheless, all of the guidelines recommend biopsy as a solving tool and a third diagnostic step in cases in which all previous examinations did not lead to a definite diagnosis of the nature of the nodules.

Both EASL/EORTC and AASLD guidelines recommend the use of percutaneous sampling in cases of atypical nodules larger than 1 cm at the end of the diagnostic algorithm, while the APASL guidelines suggest performing the procedure independently of the size of the lesions.

However, it should be considered that biopsy, affected by the risks of bleeding and seeding, might lead to a misdiagnosis in approximately 30% of the cases, mainly because of false negative results due to wrong sampling, especially in small tumors. This represents a non-negligible drawback of a method that is generally considered as a solving tool [21].

New Prospectives

Despite being very specific, the diagnosis of HCC based on the detection of the sole neoangiogenesis has shown some limitations regarding its sensitivity. Emphasized by new technological improvements, other diagnostic elements have therefore been considered [17].

Due to its intrinsic capability to assess the components of lesions also according to baseline acquisitions, such as glycogen, hemorrhage, water, or metals, and to highlight pathologic changes taking place during the carcinogenetic process, the role of MR in cirrhosis has increased continuously (fig. 3).

In fact, MR should be considered as a multiparametric technique which enables to give a paramount overview of all data that might increase the diagnostic confidence.

Two main MR tools seem to be applicable in the diagnostic work-up, i.e. diffusion-weighted imaging (DWI) and hepatocyte-specific contrast agents (fig. 4).

Diffusion-Weighted Imaging

DWI is a dedicated MR sequence which allows for the evaluation of the random motion (related to thermal effects) of water molecules ('Brownian motion') within biological tissues due to not being influenced by magnetic field strength, perfusion, or microcirculation. Its application in the abdominal district, once limited, has been possible due to the development of ultrafast sequences such as echoplanar imaging that enable the acquisition of the entire volume in a single breathholding (30–60 s per image), with a reduction of motion artefacts.

Recently, DWI has been introduced in liver MR protocols as several studies have reported its usefulness in improving the detection and characterization of focal liver lesions, especially by applying a quantitative evaluation of water molecule motion by measuring the apparent diffusion coefficient of the lesions [22].

This technique allows the detection of the restriction of water molecule diffusion within the neoplastic lesions, representing an additional element that might increase the diagnostic suspicion of a neoplasm.

Nevertheless, even if a number of studies have reported on the usefulness of DWI in differential diagnosis of benign or malignant focal liver, no consistent data are available regarding its usefulness in the differential diagnosis of a nodule within cirrhosis. Therefore, no guideline defines its role in the diagnostic algorithm [23, 24].

MR-Hepatospecific Contrast Agents

As already mentioned, intravascular contrast agents (gadolinium (Gd) chelates) allow a reliable recognition of the presence of neoangiogenesis and vascular rearrangements, which is not present in about 30% of the HCCs.

Through the progression from regenerative nodule to LGDN, to HGDN, and finally to overt HCC, a main, further parallel process takes place besides vascular alteration, represented by the progressive loss of biliary polarization of the hepatocyte and the derangement of its microscopic, secretory structure.

From a pathological point of view, it has been recently reported that two main categories of anionic, membrane transporters, represented by proteins of the family of OATP (organic anionic transporter protein) and MRP (multidrug-resistance protein), involved in the bilirubine metabolism can be altered. Those carriers are located on the sinusoidal and on the biliary pole of hepatocytes, respectively [25].

Despite no definite data are available regarding the given relationship between loss of membrane proteins and cellular dedifferentiation, especially in the case of HGDNs and early HCCs, it has been reported that membrane carriers are altered or not functioning regularly in neoplastic nodules [25]. However, both of these two preneoplastic conditions need to be carefully evaluated for a correct patient management [26].

The recent introduction of hepatobiliary contrast agents in MR studies, and especially of the highly lipophilic compound Gd-EOB-DTPA, has provided an additional tool for the assessment of the metabolic function of nodules. In fact, due to a competitive binding to bilirubine transporters, these agents allow the exploration of the residual performance of specific, hepatocytic, cellular membrane proteins and intracellular metabolic activities [27].

Moreover, these agents enable the evaluation of both dynamic vascular and metabolic nodular functions in a single-session study since the contrast is taken up within functioning hepatocytes and then excreted at the level of the biliary pole at the end of the intravascular phase. This metabolic phase occurs between 20 and 40 min after the injection; imaging acquisition of such a phase is scheduled at the end of the MR study protocol.

In recent studies, the lack of contrast agent uptake in the hepatobiliary phase has been related to a premalignant (HGDN) or malignant degeneration (early/overt HCC), even in the case of absence of the typical vascular pattern [18, 28].

Conclusions

Diagnosis of HCC still remains a challenging issue, also considering the complex management of the huge number of patients suffering from chronic liver diseases.

Surveillance is entirely focused on US examination and is otherwise affected by some limitations in terms of detection rate and specificity. In order to be characterized, nodules detected during surveillance are subject to a second-step diagnostic tool (MDCT or MR).

Until now, imaging diagnosis relies upon the detection of typical vascular patterns (wash-in/wash-out) during contrast-enhanced MDCT or MR. However, even in earlier phases of the carcinogenetic pathway, the necessity to explore different alterations that might suggest cellular dedifferentiation has been stressed.

MR has gained a major role in liver imaging due to its inherent advantages, mainly represented by the possibility to explore intracellular components, and due to new technical developments.

Therefore, a more influential role of MR by adding both DWI as well as hepatobiliary contrast agents in the diagnostic work-up can be foreseen and, consequently, a revision of the current guidelines regarding the diagnostic algorithm of HCC should be taken into consideration.

Disclosure Statement

The authors have nothing to disclose.

References

1 Davila JA, Morgan RO, Shaib Y, McGlynn KA, El-Serag HB: Hepatitis C infection and the increasing incidence of hepatocellular carcinoma: a population-based study. Gastroenterology 2004;127: 1372–1380.

2 Ascha MS, Hanouneh IA, Lopez R, Tamimi TA, Feldstein AF, Zein NN: The incidence and risk factors of hepatocellular carcinoma in patients with nonalcoholic steatohepatitis. Hepatology 2010;51: 1972–1978.

3 European Association for the Study of the Liver; European Organisation for Research and Treatment of Cancer: EASL-EORTC clinical practice guidelines: management of hepatocellular carcinoma. J Hepatol 2012;56:908–943.

4 Bruix J, Sherman M; American Association for the Study of Liver Diseases: Management of hepatocellular carcinoma: an update. Hepatology 2011;53: 1020–1022.

5 Omata M, Lesmana LA, Tateishi R, et al: Asian Pacific Association for the Study of the Liver consensus recommendations on hepatocellular carcinoma. Hepatol Int 2010;4:439–474.

6 Bruix J, Sherman M; Practice Guidelines Committee, American Association for the Study of Liver Diseases: Management of hepatocellular carcinoma. Hepatology 2005;42:1208–1236.

7 Trevisani F, De NS, Rapaccini G, et al: Semiannual and annual surveillance of cirrhotic patients for hepatocellular carcinoma: effects on cancer stage and patient survival (Italian experience). Am J Gastroenterol 2002;97:734–744.

8 Zhang BH, Yang BH, Tang ZY: Randomized controlled trial of screening for hepatocellular carcinoma. J Cancer Res Clin Oncol 2004;130:417–422.

9 Sherman M: Surveillance for hepatocellular carcinoma and early diagnosis. Clin Liver Dis 2007;11: 817–837.

10 Sherman M: The radiological diagnosis of hepatocellular carcinoma. Am J Gastroenterol 2010;105: 610–612.

11 Singal A, Volk ML, Waljee A, et al: Meta-analysis: surveillance with ultrasound for early-stage hepatocellular carcinoma in patients with cirrhosis. Aliment Pharmacol Ther 2009;30:37–47.

12 Bolondi L: Screening for hepatocellular carcinoma in cirrhosis. J Hepatol 2003;39:1076–1084.

13 Theise ND, Park YN, Kojiro M: Dysplastic nodules and hepatocarcinogenesis. Clin Liver Dis 2002;6: 497–512.

14 International Consensus Group for Hepatocellular Neoplasia: Pathologic diagnosis of early hepatocellular carcinoma: a report of the International Consensus Group for Hepatocellular Neoplasia. Hepatology 2009;49:658–664.

15 Zech CJ, Reiser MF, Herrmann KA: Imaging of hepatocellular carcinoma by computed tomography and magnetic resonance imaging: state of the art. Dig Dis 2009;27:114–124.

16 Willatt JM, Hussain HK, Adusumilli S, Marrero JA: MR imaging of hepatocellular carcinoma in the cirrhotic liver: challenges and controversies. Radiology 2008;247:311–330.

17 Bartolozzi C, Battaglia V, Bargellini I, et al: Contrast-enhanced magnetic resonance imaging of 102 nodules in cirrhosis: correlation with histological findings on explanted livers. Abdom Imaging 2012; DOI: 10.1007/s00261-012-9952-9.

18 Forner A, Vilana R, Ayuso C, et al: Diagnosis of hepatic nodules 20 mm or smaller in cirrhosis: prospective validation of the noninvasive diagnostic criteria for hepatocellular carcinoma. Hepatology 2008;47:97–104.

19 Kim K, Kim CS, Han YM, et al: Detection of hepatocellular carcinoma: gadoxetic acid-enhanced 3-dimensional magnetic resonance imaging versus multi-detector row computed tomography. J Comput Assist Tomogr 2009;33:844–850.

20 Dietrich CF: Liver tumor characterization – comments and illustrations regarding guidelines. Ultraschall Med 2012;33(suppl 1):S22–30.

21 Bolondi L, Gaiani S, Celli N, et al: Characterization of small nodules in cirrhosis by assessment of vascularity: the problem of hypovascular hepatocellular carcinoma. Hepatology 2005;42:27–34.

22 Ichikawa T, Cederle MP, Grazioli L, Marsh W: Fibrolamellar hepatocellular carcinoma: pre- and posttherapy evaluation with CT and MR imaging. Radiology 2000;217:145–151.

23 Namimoto T, Yamashita Y, Sumi S, et al: Focal liver masses: characterization with diffusion weighted echo-planar MR imaging. Radiology 1997;204:739–744.

24 Gourtsoyianni S, Papanikolaou N, Yarmenitis S, et al: Respiratory gated diffusion-weighted imaging of the liver: value of apparent diffusion coefficient measurements in the differentiation between most commonly encountered benign and malignant focal liver lesions. Eur Radiol 2008;18:486–492.

25 Narita M, Hatano E, Arizono S, et al: Expression of OATP1B3 determines uptake of Gd-EOB-DTPA in hepatocellular carcinoma. J Gastroenterol 2009;44:793–798.

26 Yu NC, Chaudhari V, Raman SS, et al: CT and MRI improve detection of hepatocellular carcinoma, compared with ultrasound alone, in patients with cirrhosis. Clin Gastroenterol Hepatol 2011;9:161–167.

27 Kitao A, Zen Y, Matsui O, et al: Hepatocellular carcinoma: signal intensity at gadoxetic acid-enhanced MR imaging – correlation with molecular transporters and histopathologic features. Radiology 2010;256:817–826.

28 Kim SH, Kim SH, Lee J, et al: Gadoxetic acid-enhanced MRI versus triple-phase MDCT for the preoperative detection of hepatocellular carcinoma. AJR Am J Roentgenol 2009;192:1675–1681.

Viszeralmedizin
Gastrointestinal Medicine and Surgery

Übersichtsarbeit · Review Article

Viszeralmedizin 2013;29:78–83
DOI: 10.1159/000350636

Online publiziert: 12. April 2013

Histopathologie und Leberbiopsie des hepatozellulären Karzinoms

Wiebke Solaß Andrea Tannapfel

Institut für Pathologie, Ruhr-Universität Bochum, Deutschland

Schlüsselwörter
Heptozelluläres Karzinom · Diagnose · Biopsie

Zusammenfassung

Hintergrund: Das hepatozelluläre Karzinom (HCC) ist der häufigste maligne Tumor der Leber. Die Differenzierung zwischen primären Lebertumoren und Metastasen kann jedoch trotz moderner bildgebender Diagnostik mitunter Schwierigkeiten bereiten, was wiederum oftmals zu einer Diskussion über die Indikation zur Leberbiopsie führt. **Methode:** Basis dieser Arbeit ist eine selektive Literaturübersicht zum Thema «HCC». Des Weiteren erfolgte die Einbeziehung publizierter Empfehlungen und Stellungnahmen nationaler und internationaler Fachgesellschaften bezüglich der Indikation zur Leberbiopsie. Die Schlussfolgerungen werden durch die Auswertung eigener Daten ergänzt. **Ergebnisse:** Histologisch müssen die unterschiedlichen Wachstumsformen des HCC unterschieden werden und eine Abgrenzung zu präkanzerösen Läsionen und einigen Sonderformen des HCC erfolgen. Es scheint also vernünftig, immer dann zu biopsieren, wenn Zweifel an der radiologischen Diagnostik oder am klinischen Verlauf bestehen. In der Biopsie soll auch juxtaläsionelles Gewebe entnommen werden, um eine häufige Leberzirrhose zu dokumentieren. Ist eine chirurgische Resektion geplant, so kann auf die Biopsie verzichtet werden. **Schlussfolgerung:** Die Leberbiopsie erlaubt die Diagnose eines HCC, wenn die histologischen und immunhistochemischen (CD34, Zytokeratin 7 und 19, Glypican 3) Parameter eindeutig sind.

Keywords
Hepatocellular carcinoma · Diagnosis · Biopsy

Summary

Histopathology and Liver Biopsy of Hepatocellular Carcinoma

Background: Hepatocellular carcinoma (HCC) is the commonest primary liver cancer. However, differentiation between primary liver cancer and metastasis can be difficult in spite of modern radiological diagnosis. This often leads to discussions about the indication for a liver biopsy. **Method:** Summary of a selective review of the literature concerning the topic 'HCC' and 'the indications for liver biopsy', including the published recommendations and position statements of specialty societies in Germany and abroad. The conclusions are supplemented with an evaluation of the authors' own experience. **Results:** Histological analysis allows differentiation between the various architectural patterns of HCC, detection of precancerous lesions, and diagnosis of rare disease. Thus, it is reasonable to recommend a liver biopsy when in doubt regarding radiological diagnosis or the patient's history. Biopsy should also include juxtalesional tissue in order to document frequent liver cirrhosis. Indication for biopsy is abdicable when surgery has already been scheduled. **Conclusion:** Liver biopsy allows the diagnosis of HCC when histological and immunohistological parameters (CD34, cytokeratin 7 and 19, glypican 3) are univocal.

KARGER
Fax +49 761 4 52 07 14
Information@Karger.com
www.karger.com

1662-6664/13/0292-0078$38.00/0

Accessible online at:
www.karger.com/vim

Prof. Dr. med. Andrea Tannapfel
Institut für Pathologie
Ruhr-Universität Bochum
Bürkle-de-la-Camp Platz 1, 44789 Bochum, Deutschland
andrea.tannapfel@rub.de

Einleitung

Im Rahmen von klinisch-pathologischen Konferenzen wird häufig der Befund einer unklaren Raumforderung in der Leber diskutiert. In diesem Zusammenhang stellt sich oft die Frage nach der Indikation zur Leberbiopsie, da die Differenzierung zwischen primären Lebertumoren und Metastasen, trotz aller Fortschritte in der Radiologie, mitunter schwierig sein kann.

Primäre Lebertumoren können sich prinzipiell aus allen Zellelementen der Leber entwickeln. Am häufigsten entstehen primäre maligne Lebertumoren jedoch aus Hepatozyten als hepatozelluläres Karzinom (HCC), gefolgt von intrahepatischen Cholangiokarzinomen (ICC), die ihren Ausgang vom Gallengangsepithel nehmen [1].

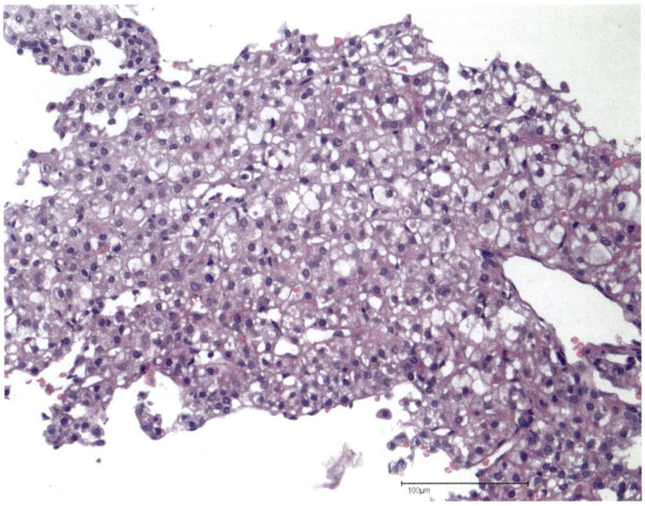

Abb. 1. HCC mit trabekulärem Wachstumsmuster und teils hellzelligen HCC-Zellen. Hämatoxylin-Eosin (HE), Maßstab im Bild.

Makroskopie

Makroskopisch zeigen HCCs hinsichtlich ihrer Farbe, Größe und Konsistenz sowie ihres Ausbreitungsmusters eine große Variationsbreite. In den meisten Fällen besteht im umgebenden Lebergewebe eine Leberzirrhose, allerdings nimmt die Inzidenz der HCCs in der nichtzirrhotischen Leber zu. Überwiegend formen HCCs unterschiedlich große, makroskopisch gelblich imponierende, teilweise grünlich aussehende, hämorrhagische Knoten, wobei die grünlich-gelbliche Farbe auf Galleninfarkte zurückzuführen ist. Die makroskopisch gelblich imponierende Erscheinungsform wird durch die zumeist vorhandene Leberzellverfettung in Kombination mit der Nekrose erklärt.

Die in der Literatur empfohlenen makroskopischen Klassifikationssysteme der HCCs nach Wachstumsformen, die 1901 von Eggel [2] vorgeschlagen wurden, unterscheiden insgesamt vier unterschiedliche Typen:

- Der expansive oder massive Typ mit einem solitären Knoten oder multiplen, scharf begrenzten Knoten (20% der Fälle).
- Der infiltrative Typ, dessen makroskopisch sichtbare Tumorgrenzen nicht eindeutig zu erkennen sind (33% der Fälle).
- Der sogenannte gemischte (expansiv und infiltrativ) Typ (42% der Fälle).
- Der diffuse Typ, in der Leberzirrhose entstanden (5% der Fälle).

Die Daten, die von Eggel publiziert wurden, basieren auf den HCCs, die in der Zirrhose entstanden sind. Allerdings ist die rein morphologische Einteilung weitestgehend verlassen worden, da sie weder Rückschlüsse auf die Ätiologie noch auf den klinischen Verlauf oder die Prognose zulässt. Besonders in zirrhotischen Lebern in fortgeschrittenen Tumorstadien besteht in etwa 50% der Fälle ein diffuses Infiltrationsmuster. Zumeist sind diese HCCs dann multifokal. Von Multifokalität wird dann gesprochen, wenn die Tumorknoten durch tumorfreies Lebergewebe voneinander getrennt sind. Satellitenknoten hingegen werden als diejenigen Knoten definiert, die kleiner sind als der Haupttumor und sich in weniger als 2 cm Entfernung von diesem befinden.

In der Literatur wird immer wieder von einem pedunkulierten HCC berichtet. Hierbei handelt es sich um ein gestieltes HCC, das aus ektopem Lebergewebe, akzessorischen Leberlappen oder unmittelbar subkapsulär gelegenen Leberabschnitten hervorgeht und in der Bildgebung extreme diagnostische Probleme bereiten kann. In den wenigen in der Literatur publizierten pedunkulierten HCCs besteht eine Verbindung zum Lebergewebe, ein sogenanntes Pedikel, jedoch werden auch Fälle beschrieben, in denen diese Verbindung zur Umgebungsleber nicht besteht. Diese Tumoren sollen eine bessere Prognose besitzen, obwohl größere Serien mit dokumentiertem Verlauf fehlen [3].

Mikroskopie

Die histologische Präsentation eines HCC reflektiert die Variabilität der Makroskopie. Es kommen unterschiedliche Wachstumsmuster vor, die auch von der Weltgesundheitsorganisation (World Health Organization, WHO) so definiert sind [4]. Am häufigsten findet sich das trabekuläre HCC (Abb. 1). Hierbei handelt es sich um Tumoren, die aus polygonalen Hepatozyten-ähnlichen Tumorzellen bestehen, die sich aus mehrschichtigen Zellbalken, sogenannten Trabekeln, zusammensetzen und sinusoidale bzw. von Endothel ausgekleidete Blutgefäße umgeben. Das pseudoglanduläre oder azinäre HCC zeigt drüsenartige Strukturen, zum Teil mit Gallebildung; auch diese Drüsen umschließen Sinusoide, die arterielles Blut führen und der Ernährung der Tumorzellen dienen (Abb. 2). Eine zirrhöse Wachstumsform des HCC zeichnet sich durch zellarme, sklerosierte, bindegewebige Septen

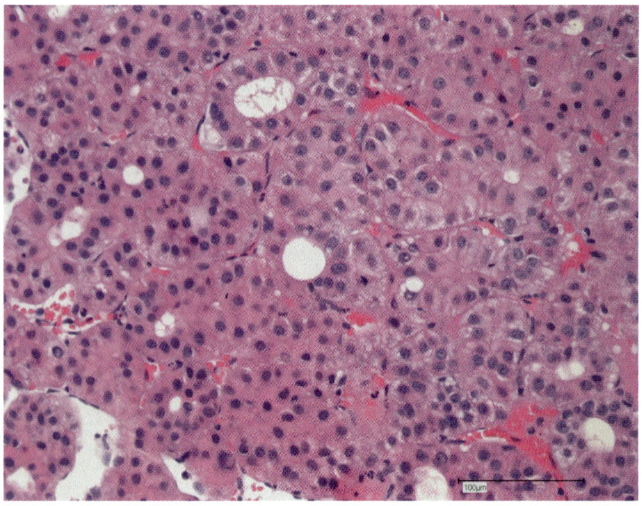

Abb. 2. Gut differenziertes HCC mit pseudoglandulärem Wachstumsmuster. Hämatoxylin-Eosin (HE), Maßstab im Bild.

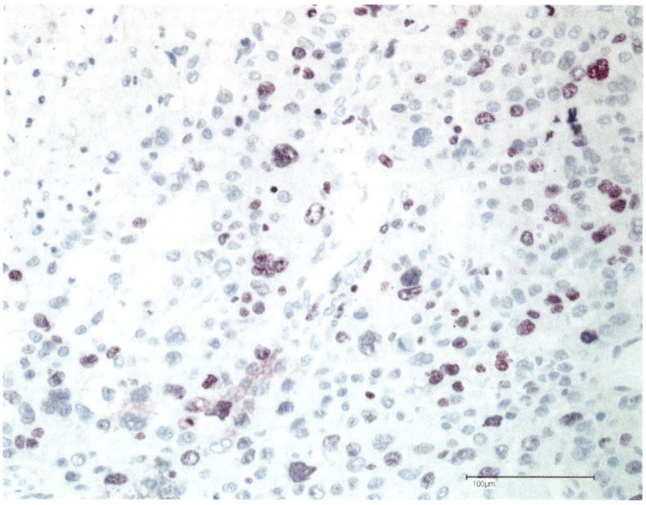

Abb. 4. Immunhistochemische Darstellung des proliferationsassoziierten Antigens MIB-1 (KI-67) in einem schlecht differenzierten HCC mit Riesenzellen (gleicher Fall wie in Abb. 3). Maßstab im Bild.

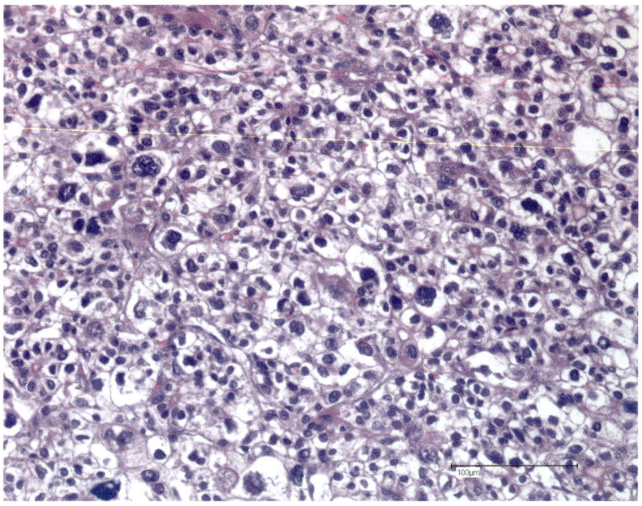

Abb. 3. Schlecht differenziertes HCC mit Riesenzellen. Hämatoxylin-Eosin (HE), Maßstab im Bild.

aus, die Tumorzellstränge umgeben, wobei hier die Tumorzellen zum Teil deutlich eosinophil erscheinen. Schlecht differenzierte HCCs zeigen ein solides oder kompaktes Wachstumsmuster ohne trabekuläre oder pseudoglanduläre Differenzierung (Abb. 3, 4).

Zytologische Varianten bestehen aus sogenannten pleomorphen Zellen, die eine große Varianz hinsichtlich der (Kern-)Größen besitzen, während Vielkernigkeit und Zellvereinzelung diese schlecht differenzierten HCCs charakterisieren. Hellzellige Tumoren zeichnen sich durch helles, glykogenreiches Zytoplasma aus. Spindelzellen zeichnen den «sarkomatoiden Typ» des HCC aus.

Nach wie vor gilt das vierstufige Grading-System für HCCs, das 1954 von Edmondson und Steiner [5] vorgeschlagen wurde. Wie bei den übrigen Organtumoren auch, basiert dieses Graduierungssystem auf unterschiedlichen zytologischen und histologischen Parametern wie Kern-Plasma-Relation, Ausmaß der Azidophilie, Chromatingehalt und Gallebildung. Die histologischen Parameter sind trabekuläre oder pseudoglanduläre Differenzierung und generell Zellkohäsivität.

Immunhistochemisch sind HCCs zumeist Zytokeratin-18-positiv, und in 30–40% der Fälle gelingt immunhistochemisch der Nachweis von Alpha-Fetoprotein (AFP).

Sonderformen des hepatozellulären Karzinoms

Fibrolamelläres Leberzellkarzinom

Das fibrolamelläre HCC macht etwa 1% aller malignen Lebertumoren aus. Zumeist sind junge Patienten, häufig Frauen, betroffen. Eine Begleitzirrhose ist in den wenigsten Fällen vorhanden. Fibrolamelläre Karzinome imponieren makroskopisch als derbe, grauweiße Tumoren, die sich relativ scharf gegen das umgebende Lebergewebe abgrenzen. Obwohl multifokales Tumorwachstum möglich ist, handelt es sich bei fibrolamellären HCCs zumeist um solitäre Herde. Interessanterweise kann im radiologischen Befund häufig eine intratumorale Verkalkung beobachtet werden [6]. Histologisch zeigen fibrolamelläre HCCs ein relativ charakteristisches Erscheinungsbild. Sie bestehen überwiegend aus bindegewebigen Stromakomponenten, während die epithelial differenzierten Tumorzellen ein feingranuliertes eosinophiles Zytoplasma zeigen, das elektronenmikroskopisch durch den hohen Gehalt an Mitochondrien begründet ist. Die bindegewebigen Septen bestehen aus dichtem azellulärem Kollagen. Die bindegewebigen Zellen umgeben die Tumorzellformationen und begründen ein charakteristisches trabekuläres oder auch umschriebenes noduläres Wachstumsmuster. Die differentialdiagnostische Abgrenzung gegenüber Cholangiokarzinomen ist hier besonders wichtig, da Cholangiokarzinome eine deutliche desmoplastische Stromareaktion besitzen können. Die Tumorzellen «mauern» sich in das Stroma ein.

Zirrhöses hepatozelluläres Karzinom

Weitere Subtypen sind das sogenannte zirrhöse hepatozelluläre Karzinom, das etwa 5% der HCCs ausmacht. Diese Tumoren zeichnen sich durch eine deutliche Fibrose aus, die Tumorzellen umgeben, die sinusoidal angeordnet sind oder trabekulär wachsen. Diese Tumoren finden sich zumeist unmittelbar unterhalb der Leberkapsel. Es ist bekannt, dass bei multifokalen HCCs durchaus ein Tumorknoten ein zirrhöses Wachstumsmuster besitzen kann. Wichtig in diesem Zusammenhang ist die differentialdiagnostische Abgrenzung gegenüber Cholangiokarzinomen und dem fibrolamellären Karzinom.

Undifferenziertes Karzinom

Das undifferenzierte Karzinom zeichnet sich dadurch aus, dass es keine Wachstumsrichtung vorweist; lediglich die Zytokeratin-Immunhistochemie zeigt an, dass es sich um ein Karzinom handelt. Undifferenzierte Leberzellkarzinome sind selten und machen weniger als 2% aller epithelialen Lebertumoren aus.

Lymphoepitheliales Karzinom

Das lymphoepitheliale Karzinom ist ein pleomorpher Tumor, der – wie bei anderen lymphoepithelialen Karzinomen und anderen Organen ebenfalls – eine ausgeprägte Lymphozyteninfiltration aufweist. Die Tumorzellen sind charakteristischerweise positiv gegenüber Bestandteilen des Epstein-Barr-Virus.

Sarkomatoides hepatozelluläres Karzinom

Das sarkomatoide HCC besteht aus Spindelzellen, die an ein Sarkom erinnern. Immunhistochemisch zeigt sich allerdings eine Zytokeratin-Expression, sodass eine Unterscheidung zu einem Sarkom als mesenchymaler Tumor ohne Zytokeratin-Expression erfolgen kann.

Präkanzeröse Läsionen und Differentialdiagnostik

Vorläuferläsionen sind dysplastische Knoten, die sich grundsätzlich nur in Zirrhoselebern finden. In seltenen Fällen könnten sie Folge von schweren chronischen Leberschädigungen (z.B. nach Paracetamol-Intoxikation) sein [7]. Definitionsgemäß sind dysplastische Knoten kleiner als 1 cm, in einigen Serien kleiner als 0,5 cm. Dysplastische Knoten werden abhängig von Art und Ausmaß der zellulären Atypien als niedriggradig oder hochgradig dysplastische Knoten graduiert. Dysplastische Knoten müssen von fokalen nodulären Hyperplasien, Leberzelladenomen und nodulär regenerativen Hyperplasien abgegrenzt werden. Die Terminologie eines «frühen» HCC wird in der internationalen Literatur zwar häufig – insbesondere im asiatischen Raum – verwendet, ist allerdings hinsichtlich der Histologie der Tumoren schwierig zu reproduzieren.

«Frühe» HCCs sind unscharf begrenzte Knoten, die meist kleiner als 2 cm sind und mikroskopisch aus gut differenzierten HCC-Zellen bestehen. Histologisch fällt eine erhöhte zelluläre Dichte auf, das Wachstumsmuster wird unregelmäßig, pseudoglanduläre Strukturen und degenerative Veränderungen der Zellen mit Verfettung können sichtbar sein. Alle histologischen Kennzeichen, die für ein frühes HCC typisch sind, können auch in fortgeschrittenen HCCs (größer als 2 cm) festgestellt werden [8].

Als einziges sicheres Unterscheidungsmerkmal zwischen frühem und fortgeschrittenem HCC gilt das Kriterium der Gefäßversorgung. Frühe HCCs zeigen portale Gefäße und eine unterschiedliche Anzahl von unpaaren, zum Teil wandaufbaugestörten arteriellen Gefäßen. Fortgeschrittene HCCs zeigen definitionsgemäß keine portalen Gefäße und eine gut entwickelte arterielle Versorgung aus unpaaren arteriellen Gefäßstrukturen. Allerdings ist diese Unterscheidung in Leberbiopsien oder in Resektaten ohne immunhistochemische Aufarbeitung nicht immer möglich. Da sich hieraus keine therapeutische Konsequenz ergibt, ist die Unterscheidung im klinischen Alltag verzichtbar.

Aufgrund der ausgesprochen großen histologischen Variabilität von primären malignen Lebertumoren kann die Diagnose eines HCC bzw. die Abgrenzung gegenüber Metastasen eines Adenokarzinoms oder auch eines malignen neuroendokrinen Tumors in der Leber schwierig sein. Während gut differenzierte HCCs zumeist relativ einfach zu diagnostizieren sind, muss hier lediglich die Abgrenzung zu Leberzelladenomen erfolgen; die Diagnose kann bei schlecht differenzierten, solide wachsenden HCCs jedoch sehr schwierig sein. Relativ typisch für HCCs sind zytologische Kriterien wie eosinophiles Zytoplasma, eosinophile intrazytoplasmatische Einschlusskörper, histologisch sinusoidale Auskleidung der Tumorzellnester und Gallebildung. Ein weiteres wichtiges differentialdiagnostisches Kriterium ist die Beobachtung, dass HCCs in Zirrhose fast nie die Sinusoide des umgebenden nichtneoplastischen Lebergewebes infiltrierten – ganz im Gegensatz zu Metastasen in der Leber oder primären Cholangiokarzinomen.

Leberbiopsie: Warum und wann?

Die perkutane, sonographisch kontrollierte Leberpunktion ist weltweit der Goldstandard für die Diagnose von Lebertumoren, jedoch bleibt häufig die Frage der Indikationsstellung. Generell muss der Stellenwert der Leberbiopsie bei fokalen Leberläsionen individuell diskutiert werden, sodass eine pauschale Empfehlung nicht gegeben werden kann. Es gilt jedoch, dass repräsentative Leberbiopsien im klinischen Alltag bei mehr als 90% der Fälle die definitive Diagnosestellung ermöglichen [9].

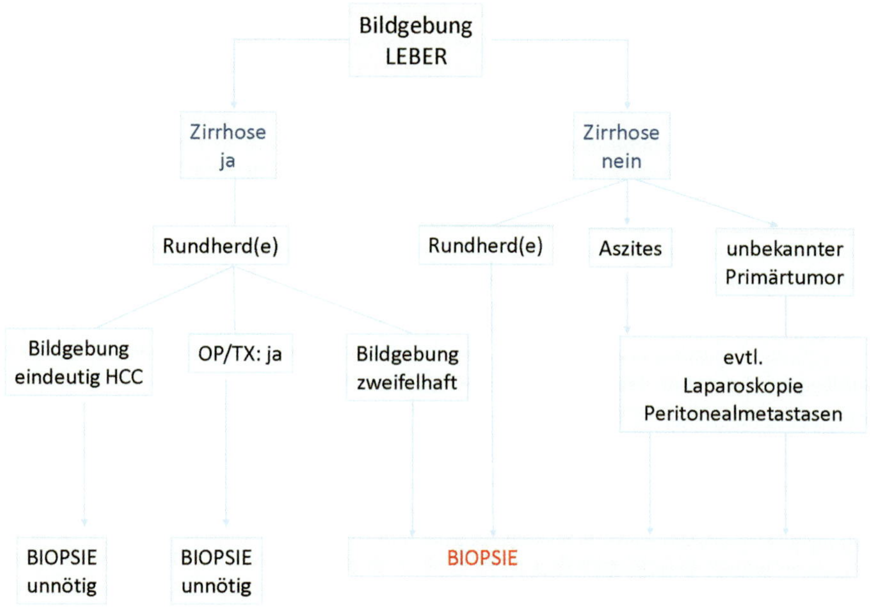

Abb. 5. Entscheidungspfad für die Biopsie.

Die internationalen Empfehlungen zur Leberbiopsie bei fokalen Leberläsionen sind lediglich bei Rundherden in nichtzirrhotischer Leber eindeutig. Es wird empfohlen, solitäre Leberläsionen ohne bekannte Leberzirrhose zu biopsieren. In dieser Situation (nichtzirrhotische Leber) ist die Abgrenzung von gut differenzierten HCCs zu Leberzelladenomen oder intrahepatischen Cholangiokarzinomen mitunter schwierig.

Nach neueren Literaturdaten wird das Leberzelladenom als Neubildung von terminal differenzierten Hepatozyten verstanden. Man weiß heute, dass das Leberzelladenom keine homogene Entität darstellt, sondern mindestens drei unterschiedliche molekularpathologisch definierte Neoplasien darstellen kann [10]. Etwa 30–40% der Leberzelladenome entstehen bei Frauen, sind mit einer Steatosis hepatis assoziiert und besitzen die klassische Histologie eines Leberzelladenoms. Molekularbiologisch sind diese Leberzelladenome durch eine Inaktivierung von HNF-1α charakterisiert. 40% der Leberzelladenome sind sogenannte inflammatorische oder teleangiektatische Leberzelladenome, die bei Frauen und Männern gleich häufig vorkommen sowie mit einer nichtalkoholischen Fettlebererkrankung (Non-Alcoholic Fatty Liver Disease, NAFLD), einem metabolischen Syndrom oder einer Alkoholanamnese assoziiert sind. 10% der Leberzelladenome sind durch eine β-Catenin-Inaktivierung entstanden, treten häufig bei Männern auf und ähneln zytologisch einem HCC. Bei diesen Leberzelladenomen ist die maligne Transformationswahrscheinlichkeit erhöht. Derzeit wird diskutiert, ob es sich bei dieser Subgruppe möglicherweise schon um HCCs handelt.

Die internationalen Empfehlungen zur Biopsie von Rundherden in Zirrhoseleber sind heterogen. Die Amerikanische Fachgesellschaft zum Studium der Leber (American Association for the Study of Liver Diseases, AASLD) gibt eine differenzierte Empfehlung. Wenn die Knoten, die sonographisch oder CT-morphologisch in der zirrhotischen Leber dargestellt wurden, kleiner als 1 cm sind, ist eine Biopsie nicht notwendig; eine Verlaufskontrolle soll nach 3–4 Monaten vorgenommen werden. Ist die Läsion größer als 1 cm (oder größenprogredient), dann soll eine radiologische Bildgebung ergänzt werden. Bei typischem Befund in zwei unterschiedlichen radiologischen Verfahren soll die weitere Therapie wie beim HCC erfolgen; eine Leberbiopsie ist dann überflüssig. Erzielen die beiden unabhängigen radiologischen Befunde aber kein eindeutiges Ergebnis, sollte hingegen eine Biopsie durchgeführt werden (Abb. 5).

In diesem Zusammenhang ist es von Bedeutung, dass insbesondere Läsionen, die kleiner als 2 cm im Durchmesser sind, eine duale Blutperfusion besitzen können, sodass die radiologischen Kriterien (arterielle Perfusion, venöser Abstrom) hier keine Gültigkeit besitzen. Die bildmorphologisch nachweisbare Perfusion von dysplastischen Knoten ist in unterschiedlichen Publikationen divergent bewertet. Zusammenfassend können dysplastische Knoten ein sehr heterogenes Durchblutungsmuster besitzen und entziehen sich damit der definitiven radiologischen Diagnose. Leider sind dysplastische Knoten auch durch eine Leberbiopsie kaum von HCCs abzugrenzen, sodass in dieser Situation ein interdisziplinäres, klinisch abgestimmtes Verhalten anzuraten ist.

Die Differenzierung in ein «kleines» HCC oder «Carcinoma in situ» in der japanischen Literatur ist klinisch irrelevant, da die therapeutischen Konsequenzen unabhängig von diesen diagnostischen, von der WHO nicht definierten Entitäten erfolgen. In jedem Fall muss eine Intervention erfolgen, ob es sich um ein kleines HCC, um ein Carcinoma in situ oder um einen sogenannten dysplastischen Knoten handelt.

Alle internationalen und nationalen Leitlinien sind sich einig, dass die Indikation zur Leberbiopsie beim Verdacht auf

HCC unabhängig vom Serum/AFP-Wert gestellt werden soll. Aufgrund von nachweisbaren AFP-Werterhöhungen bei aktiver Zirrhose bzw. Cholestase oder auch bei AFP-Werterhöhung bei intrahepatischen Cholangiokarzinomen wird die Spezifität des AFP-Wertes inzwischen kritisch gesehen. Daher spielt der AFP-Wert in der Diagnostik des HCC bzw. der Indikation zur Biopsie keine wesentliche Rolle mehr.

Gegen eine Leberbiopsie sprechen die verfahrensbedingten Komplikationen, insbesondere die Nachblutung und die Tumorzellverschleppung. In großen Studien werden signifikante Blutungskomplikationen bei etwa 1% der Leberbiopsien dokumentiert, wobei die Mortalität unter 0,1% liegt. Das Risiko einer Nachblutung ist bei diffusen Leberprozessen, wie z.B. Lymphomen, deutlich höher als bei primären malignen Lebertumoren.

Die in der Literatur publizierte Prävalenz von sogenannten Stichkanalmetastasen schwankt von 0,0095 bis 5% [11]. Allerdings sind die meisten diesbezüglichen Studien retrospektiv, die Stichkanalmetastasen nicht histologisch gesichert, und eine Abgrenzung zu Zweittumoren (intrahepatische HCC-Metastasen) erfolgt nicht. Auch werden heterogene Patienten innerhalb dieser Studien miteinander verglichen. Zumeist wird nicht differenziert, ob fortgeschrittene oder frühe Tumorstadien vorliegen, Aszites besteht oder beispielsweise mehrere Tumorknoten bereits vorliegen. Es ist also schwierig, diese Daten in schlüssiger Form zusammenzufassen; jedoch wird heute von einer generellen Inzidenz von Stichkanalmetastasen von 2,7% ausgegangen. Die Prognose der Patienten mit Stichkanalmetastasen wird durch diese Komplikation nicht bestimmt: In den veröffentlichten Serien versterben die Patienten nicht an den Stichkanalmetastasen, sondern an den Folgen ihrer systemischen Tumorerkrankung.

Patienten mit kompensierter Leberzirrhose sind keine Kandidaten für eine Lebertransplantation, solange sie kein HCC aufweisen. Aus diesem Grund soll die Diagnose eines HCC gesichert werden, bevor der Patient in die Transplantationsliste aufgenommen wird. Auch in dieser klinischen Situation sind die diagnostischen Kriterien der AASLD gültig [12]. Besteht klinisch und/oder radiologisch noch ein Zweifel über die Diagnose eines HCC, so soll eine Leberbiopsie vorgenommen werden. Das Risiko einer Leberbiopsie für eine hämatogene Tumorzelldissemination bei transplantierten Patienten wurde nicht abschließend evaluiert. Es gibt jedoch keine klare Evidenz, dass das Rezidivrisiko eines HCC nach Lebertransplantation durch eine Leberbiopsie erhöht ist. Aus diesen Gründen ist eine frühere Leberbiopsie keine Kontraindikation für eine Lebertransplantation [13].

Nach Wertung aller nationalen und internationalen Überlegungen scheint es vernünftig, bei Verdacht auf HCC die Läsion und das juxtaläsionelle Gewebe immer dann zu biopsieren, wenn Zweifel an der radiologischen Diagnostik oder am klinischen Verlauf bestehen. Ein HCC ist dann sicher zu diagnostizieren, wenn die histologischen und immunhistochemischen Parameter (CD34, Zytokeratin 7 und 19, Glypican 3) eindeutig sind. Zudem erlaubt die Leberbiopsie eine Aussage über eine vorliegende Leberzirrhose und deren Ätiologie [14]. Grundsätzlich kann auf eine Biopsie verzichtet werden, wenn die Indikation zur chirurgischen Resektion schon gestellt wurde [15]. Der Status des Umgebungslebergewebes (Staging und Grading der Zirrhose) ist allerdings bei der präoperativen Bestimmung des zulässigen Resektionsausmaßes oft hilfreich.

Disclosure Statement

Prof. Tannapfel erhielt Honorare für Beratertätigkeit von den Firmen Merck, Sanofi, Falk, Pfizer, Amgen, AstraZeneca, Lilly und Novartis. Reisekostenerstattung und Vortragshonorare bekam sie von den Firmen Sanofi, Falk, Pfizer, Amgen und Apda.

Dr. Solaß bestätigt, dass sie keine Interessenkonflikte hat.

Literatur

1 Tischoff I, Tannapfel A: Hepatocellular carcinoma and cholangiocarcinoma – different prognosis, pathogenesis and therapy. Zentralbl Chir 2007;132: 300–305.

2 Eggel H: Über das primäre Carcinom der Leber. Beitr Pathol Anat Allg Pathol 1901;30:506–604.

3 Yeh CN, Lee WC, Jeng LB, Chen MF: Pedunculated hepatocellular carcinoma: clinicopathologic study of 18 surgically resected cases. World J Surg 2002;26:1133–1138.

4 Bosman FT, Carneiro F, Hruban RH (eds): WHO Classification of Tumours of the Digestive System, vol 3. Geneva, IARC World Health Organ, 2010.

5 Edmondson HA, Steiner PE: Primary carcinoma of the liver: a study of 100 cases among 48,900 necropsies. Cancer 1954;7:462–503.

6 Chun YS, Zimmitti G: Fibrolamellar variant of hepatocellular carcinoma. Recent Results Cancer Res 2013;190:101–110.

7 Park YN: Update on precursor and early lesions of hepatocellular carcinomas. Arch Pathol Lab Med 2011;135:704–715.

8 Roncalli M, Terracciano L, Di Tommaso L, David E, Colombo M; Gruppo Italiano Patologi Apparato Digerente (GIPAD); Società Italiana di Anatomia Patologica e Citopatologia Diagnostica/International Academy of Pathology, Italian division (SIAPEC/IAP): Liver precancerous lesions and hepatocellular carcinoma: the histology report. Dig Liver Dis 2011;43(suppl 4):S361–372.

9 Tannapfel A, Dienes HP, Lohse AW: The indications for liver biopsy. Dtsch Arztebl Int 2012;109: 477–483.

10 van Aalten SM, Witjes CD, de Man RA, Ijzermans JN, Terkivatan T: Can a decision-making model be justified in the management of hepatocellular adenoma? Liver Int 2012;32:28–37.

11 Silva MA, Hegab B, Hyde C, Guo B, Buckels JA, Mirza DF: Needle track seeding following biopsy of liver lesions in the diagnosis of hepatocellular cancer: a systematic review and meta-analysis. Gut 2008;57:1592–1596.

12 Sherman M: The radiological diagnosis of hepatocellular carcinoma. Am J Gastroenterol 2010;105: 610–612.

13 Durand F, Belghiti J, Paradis V: Liver transplantation for hepatocellular carcinoma: role of biopsy. Liver Transpl 2007;13(suppl 2):S17–23.

14 Stölzel U, Tannapfel A: Indications for liver biopsy in liver tumors. Zentralbl Chir 2000;125: 606–609.

15 Cho SW, Marsh JW, Steel J, Holloway SE, Heckman JT, Ochoa ER, Geller DA, Gamblin TC: Surgical management of hepatocellular adenoma: take it or leave it? Ann Surg Oncol 2008;15: 2795–2803.

Viszeralmedizin
Gastrointestinal Medicine and Surgery

Übersichtsarbeit · Review Article

Viszeralmedizin 2013;29:84–91
DOI: 10.1159/000351067

Online publiziert: 12. April 2013

Systemische Therapie des hepatozellulären Karzinoms

Martha M. Kirstein Arndt Vogel

Abteilung für Gastroenterologie, Hepatologie und Endokrinologie, Medizinische Hochschule Hannover, Deutschland

Schlüsselwörter
Hepatozeluläres Karzinom · Sorafenib · c-MET · Tivantinib

Zusammenfassung
Hintergrund: Das hepatozelluläre Karzinom (HCC) ist eine der häufigsten Tumorerkrankungen weltweit. Mit dem Multikinase-Inhibitor Sorafenib konnte erstmals ein signifikanter Überlebensvorteil bei Patienten mit fortgeschrittenem HCC gezeigt werden. Bis heute ist Sorafenib die einzige zugelassene systemisch wirksame Substanz für Patienten mit fortgeschrittenem HCC. Die weiteren Behandlungsoptionen für Patienten mit einem fortgeschrittenen HCC sind jedoch beschränkt. Es fehlen insbesondere Second-line-Therapien für Patienten, die Sorafenib nicht tolerieren und/oder hierunter progredient werden. **Methode:** Neue molekulare Therapien befinden sich in klinischer Entwicklung, bislang allerdings mit zumeist ernüchternden Ergebnissen. **Ergebnisse:** Untersuchungen der alternativen Angiogenese-Inhibitoren Sunitinib und Brivanib, der EGFR(epidermaler Wachstumsfaktor-Rezeptor)-Inhibitoren Erlotinib, Gefitinib, Lapatinib und Cetuximab sowie des MEK(Mitogen-aktivierte Proteinkinase)-Inhibitors Selumetinib waren bislang nicht zielführend. Erfolg versprechend erscheint die Inhibition von c-MET mit Tivantinib, die bei c-MET-überexprimierenden Patienten eine signifikante Verlängerung des Überlebens und der Zeit zur Progression erbrachte. Untersuchungen von anderen Zielgruppen wie unter anderem Inhibitoren von mTOR, PI3K/Akt und IGFR befinden sich in teils noch früher klinischer Entwicklung und bleiben abzuwarten. **Schlussfolgerungen:** Die Entwicklung der systemischen Behandlung des HCC bleibt anspruchsvoll. Zunehmend zeichnet sich ab, dass bei HCC-Patienten eine schwierige Balance zwischen Toxizität der Behandlung und antitumoraler Wirkung besteht, die eine signifikante Verbesserung des Überlebens der Patienten ermöglicht. Eine Lösung dieses Dilemmas könnte in der Identifikation von prognostischen und prädiktiven Faktoren wie c-MET bestehen, die eine personalisierte und effektive Therapie in Subgruppen der HCC-Patienten ermöglichen sollte.

Keywords
Hepatocellular carcinoma · Sorafenib · c-MET · Tivantinib

Summary
Systemic Therapy for Hepatocellular Carcinoma
Background: Hepatocellular carcinoma (HCC) is one of the most common and deadly malignancies worldwide. The multikinase inhibitor sorafenib has provided a survival benefit in patients with advanced HCC. Sorafenib remains the only approved agent for advanced HCC. There are only few systemic therapeutic options. No standardized second-line treatment exists for patients with progressive disease during sorafenib treatment or with intolerable side effects. **Method:** Novel molecular targets are under clinical development, with sobering outcomes so far. **Results:** Investigations of the alternative inhibitors of angiogenesis, i.e. sunitinib and brivanib, the EGFR (epidermal growth factor receptor) inhibitors erlotinib, gefitinib, lapatinib, and cetuximab as well as the MEK (mitogen-activated protein kinase) inhibitor selumetinib did not provide constructive results. Targeting c-MET with the associated inhibitor tivantinib appears to be a promising option. Overall survival and time to progression was significantly prolonged with tivantinib in patients overexpressing c-MET. Moreover, targets such as mTOR, PI3K/Akt, and IGFR, among others, are under clinical development, though partially in early stages. The results remain to be seen. **Conclusions:** Systemic management of HCC remains challenging. Among HCC patients, a difficult balance between the toxicity of the treatment and the antitumoral effect can be ascertained, enabling a significant improvement of the survival of the patients. There is an urgent need for the identification of predictive and prognostic factors such as C-MET for a personalized and efficient treatment in subgroups of HCC patients.

KARGER
Fax +49 761 4 52 07 14
Information@Karger.com
www.karger.com

1662-6664/13/0292-0084$38.00/0

Accessible online at:
www.karger.com/vim

Prof. Dr. med. Arndt Vogel
Abteilung für Gastroenterologie, Hepatologie und Endokrinologie
Medizinische Hochschule Hannover
Carl-Neuberg-Straße 1, 30625 Hannover, Deutschland
Vogel.Arndt@mh-hannover.de

Einleitung

Das hepatozelluläre Karzinom (HCC) ist weltweit der siebthäufigste Tumor (am fünfthäufigsten bei Männern, am achthäufigsten bei Frauen) [1]. Aufgrund der immer noch unzureichenden Behandlungsoptionen für Patienten im fortgeschrittenen Tumorstadium ist das HCC die dritthäufigste tumorvermittelte Todesursache (*www.iarc.fr*). 2008 waren entsprechend der schlechten Prognose dieser Tumorerkrankung bei 748 300 Neuerkrankungen 695 900 Todesfälle zu verzeichnen.

Das HCC entsteht in 70–80% aller Fälle auf dem Boden einer Leberzirrhose, die die Funktion der Leber in der Regel deutlich beeinträchtigt. Komplikationen der Leberzirrhose wie Blutungen aus Ösophagusvarizen, Aszites oder eine hepatische Enzephalopathie tragen zur hohen Mortalität und Morbidität der Patienten bei. Das über 5 Jahre kumulierte Risiko von zirrhotischen Patienten, ein HCC zu entwickeln, liegt zwischen 5 und 30% [1]. Die hauptsächlichen Risikofaktoren für die Entstehung einer Leberzirrhose und damit eines HCC sind chronische Infektionen mit dem Hepatitis-B-Virus (HBV) oder Hepatitis-C-Virus (HCV) und Alkoholabusus. Zudem wird das HCC-Risiko durch nicht alkoholbedingte Leberverfettung (nonalcoholic fatty liver disease, NAFLD; nonalcoholic steatohepatitis, NASH) erhöht. Hinzu kommen seltenere Risikofaktoren wie Hämochromatose, Tyrosinämie, Autoimmunhepatitis, einige Porphyrien und Morbus Wilson. Diabetes, Adipositas, Rauchen, männliches Geschlecht und fortgeschrittenes Alter erhöhen zusätzlich das Risiko, an einem HCC zu erkranken.

Die «Barcelona Clinic Liver Cancer (BCLC)»-Klassifikation ist das gegenwärtig am häufigsten verwendete Staging-System und gibt für jedes Stadium orientierende therapeutische Empfehlungen [2–3]. Allerdings muss die individuelle Therapieempfehlung jedes HCC-Patienten in einem interdisziplinären Tumorboard getroffen werden. Die BCLC-Klassifikation unterscheidet zwischen fünf Stadien des HCC (BCLC-0 sowie BCLC-A bis BCLC-D) und bezieht dabei den Tumorstatus, die Leberfunktion und den allgemeinen Gesundheitszustand der Patienten ein. Grundsätzlich kann man nach therapeutischer Zielsetzung in ein Stadium mit kurativen (BCLC-0 und BCLC-A) und palliativen (BCLC-B bis BCLC-D) Optionen (Abb. 1) differenzieren.

Bis vor wenigen Jahren gab es bis auf bestmögliche unterstützende Maßnahmen (Best Supportive Care) keine palliative Behandlungsmöglichkeit für Patienten, die einer lokoregionalen Therapie nicht zugänglich waren. Herkömmliche Chemotherapien können zum einen durch die zumeist zugrunde liegende Leberzirrhose und die damit einhergehende Thrombozytopenie/Panzytopenie nicht eingesetzt werden. Zum anderen ist das HCC auch weitestgehend resistent gegen traditionelle Chemotherapien. Dies änderte sich mit der Verfügbarkeit des oralen Multikinase-Inhibitors Sorafenib, der sowohl die Tumorangiogenese als auch die Tumorproliferation und damit zwei charakteristische Stoffwechselwege des stark vaskularisierten HCC hemmt. Seine Angriffspunkte sind die Rezeptor-Tyrosinkinasen VEGFR 1–3, PDGF-β, Flt-3 und c-Kit, die am Anfang intrazellulärer Phosphorylierungskaskaden stehen und die Gefäßversorgung des Tumors vermitteln. Darüber hinaus inhibiert Sorafenib das Raf-Protein, ein Schlüsselmolekül des Mitogen-aktivierten Proteinkinase-Signalwegs (MAPK), der eine zentrale Rolle bei der Zellproliferation spielt. Für die europäischen Fachgesellschaften repräsentiert Sorafenib in ihren aktuellen Richtlinien die einzige HCC-Therapie von gleichzeitig höchstem Evidenzlevel und Empfehlungsgrad. Nichtsdestotrotz ist der klinische

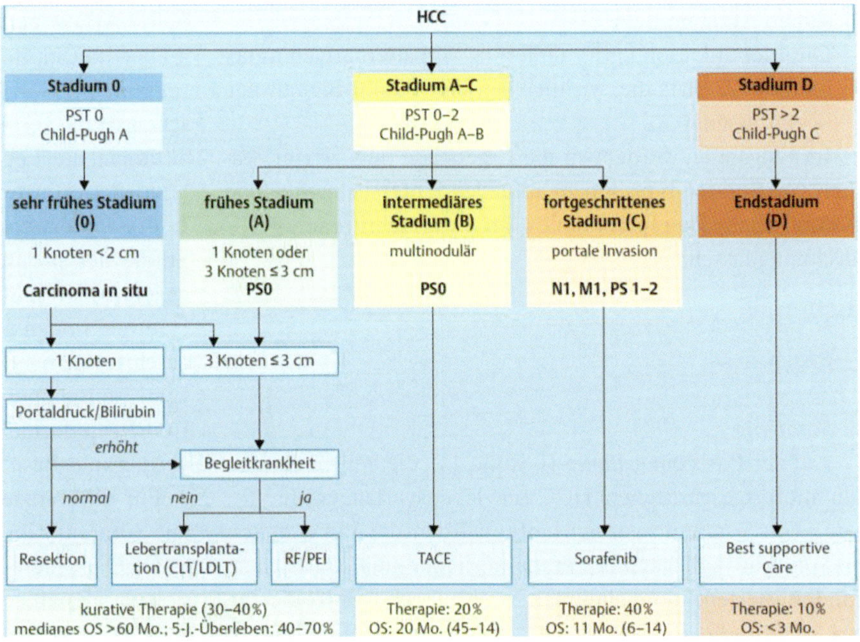

Abb. 1. Einteilung der Stadien und Behandlung nach der BCLC-Klassifikation (PST = Performance-Status, RF/PEI = Radiofrequenzablation/perkutane Ethanolinjektion, TACE = transarterielle Chemoembolisation) (aus [38], mit freundlicher Genehmigung des Georg Thieme Verlags, Stuttgart; modifiziert nach [2]).

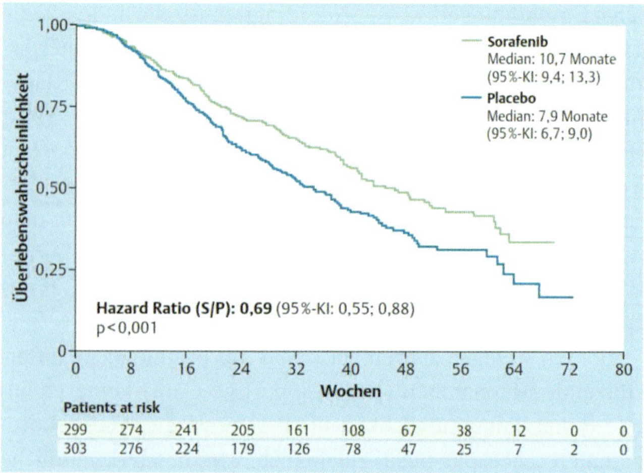

Abb. 2. Sorafenib bei Patienten mit fortgeschrittenem HCC: Gesamtüberleben (aus [38], mit freundlicher Genehmigung des Georg Thieme Verlags, Stuttgart; modifiziert nach [5]).

Benefit von Sorafenib leider nur begrenzt, und die Behandlungsoptionen des fortgeschrittenen HCC müssen dringend verbessert und erweitert werden.

Die Zulassung von Sorafenib führte zu einem starken Anstoß der Arzneimittelentwicklung im HCC-Bereich. Eine große Anzahl verschiedener molekularer Substanzen, die in bekannte Signalwege der Hepatokarzinogenese eingreifen oder auch gegen neue Zielmoleküle gerichtet sind, befinden sich derzeit in unterschiedlichen Phasen der klinischen Entwicklung. Hierbei lassen sich prinzipiell drei Vorgehensweisen unterscheiden:

- Die Kombination von Sorafenib mit bekannten, antiproliferativ und/oder antiangiogenetisch wirksamen Arzneimitteln.
- Die Testung von alternativen, antiangiogenetisch wirksamen Arzneimitteln.
- Die Identifikation und Validierung von alternativen molekularen Zielen, die wichtige andere Tumor-Signalwege beeinflussen.

Im Folgenden werden wir die Ergebnisse publizierter Studien von Sorafenib bis hin zu aktuellen Untersuchungen von systemischen Therapieoptionen im fortgeschrittenen HCC zusammenfassen.

Ergebnisse

Sorafenib

Auf der Basis einer Phase-II-Studie [4], die bei 137 Patienten mit fortgeschrittenem HCC eine lebensverlängernde Wirkung von Sorafenib gezeigt hatte, wurden die Wirksamkeit und die Verträglichkeit des Präparats in der multizentrischen, randomisierten, doppelblinden und placebokontrollierten SHARP-Studie (Sorafenib HCC Assessment Randomized Protocol Trial) geprüft [5]. Diese Phase-III-Studie schloss 602 Patienten in 121 Behandlungszentren aus 21 Ländern (Europäische Union/EU, Nord- und Südamerika, Australien) mit überwiegend fortgeschrittenem HCC ein (18% der Sorafenib- und 17% der Placebo-Gruppe befanden sich erst im intermediären Stadium BCLC-B). Weitere Einschlusskriterien waren eine gut erhaltene Leberfunktion (Child-Pugh A), ein ECOG-Performance-Status von höchstens 2 und eine Lebenserwartung von mindestens 12 Wochen. 299 Patienten wurden in den Sorafenib-Arm (400 mg peroral 2-mal täglich) und 303 Patienten in den Placebo-Arm der Studie randomisiert.

Bereits nach der zweiten Interimsanalyse wurde die Studie abgebrochen, weil sich signifikante Überlebensvorteile in der Sorafenib-Gruppe zeigten (Abb. 2). Die mediane Gesamtüberlebenszeit unter Sorafenib betrug 10,7 Monate gegenüber 7,9 Monaten in der Placebo-Gruppe (Hazard Ratio (HR) 0,69; 95%-Konfidenzintervall (KI) 0,55–0,87; p = 0,00058). Sorafenib verbesserte auch die mittlere Zeit bis zur radiologisch ermittelten Tumorprogression von 2,8 auf 5,5 Monate (HR 0,58; 95%-KI 0,44–0,74; p = 0,000007). Kein statistisch signifikanter Unterschied zwischen beiden Gruppen ergab sich hinsichtlich der ermittelten Zeit bis zur symptomatischen Progression (4,1 vs. 4,9 Monate; HR 1,08; 95%-KI 0,88–1,31; p = 0,77). Sorafenib zeigte in allen Subgruppen einen Vorteil im Gesamtüberleben gegenüber Placebo [6–9].

Die Ergebnisse der SHARP-Studie veranlassten die europäische und die amerikanische Arzneimittelbehörde, Sorafenib Ende 2007 als erstes Medikament zur Behandlung des HCC (EU) bzw. des nicht resezierbaren HCC (USA) zuzulassen.

In der SHARP-Studie wurde eine Behandlungsunterbrechung aufgrund von Nebenwirkungen bei 38% der mit Sorafenib behandelten Patienten gegenüber 37% der Patienten in der Kontrollgruppe notwendig. Die meisten Nebenwirkungen waren dermatologischer, gastrointestinaler und konstitutioneller Art, wobei die häufigsten Toxizitäten vom Grad 3 oder 4 Diarrhö (Sorafenib 8%, Placebo 2%) und Hand-Fuß-Hautreaktionen (Sorafenib 8%, Placebo <1%) waren. Im klinischen Alltag vermindern insbesondere die Hand-Fuß-Hautreaktionen die Lebensqualität deutlich und führen häufig zu Unterdosierungen oder Therapieunterbrechungen (Abb. 3). Interessanterweise konnte in einer großen randomisierten Studie der prophylaktische Effekt harnstoffhaltiger Salben gegenüber Best Supportive Care bei Patienten mit Hand-Fuß-Hautreaktionen unter der Behandlung mit Sorafenib bei fortgeschrittenem HCC gezeigt werden, sodass analog zur präventiven Behandlung von Patienten mit Kolonkarzinom unter EGFR(epidermaler Wachstumsfaktor-Rezeptor)-Antikörpertherapie diese auch bei HCC-Patienten erfolgen kann [10].

Für differenziertere Aufschlüsse über die HCC-Therapie mit Sorafenib im klinischen Alltag wurden im Rahmen der GIDEON-Studie (Global Investigation of Therapeutic Decisions in Hepatocellular Carcinoma and of its Treatment with Sorafenib) 2770 Patienten aus 37 Ländern (37% EU) zwi-

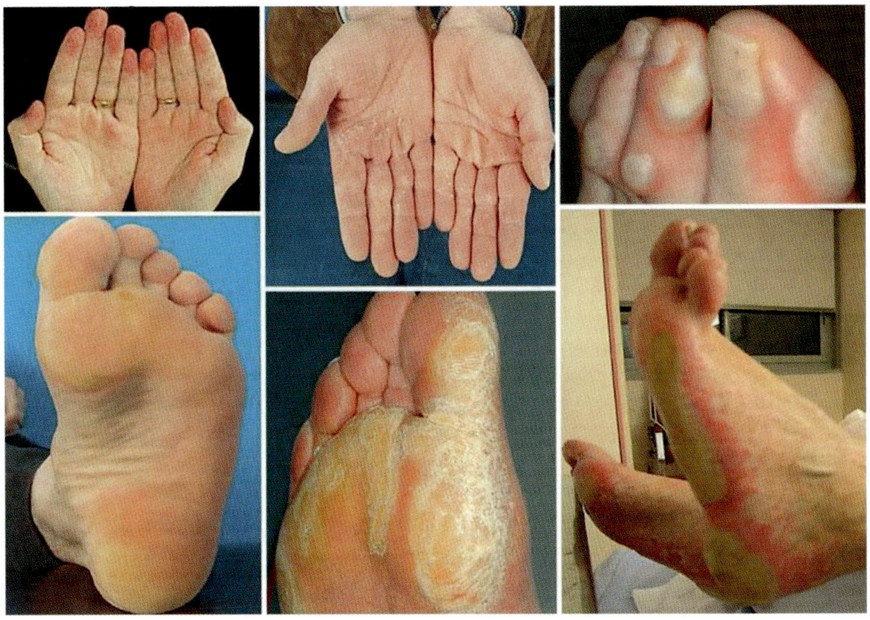

Abb. 3. Der Preis der Therapie: Das Hand-Fuß-Syndrom unter der Behandlung mit Sorafenib (aus [39]; Copyright S. Karger AG, Basel).

schen Januar 2009 und Dezember 2010 für eine systemische Therapie mit Sorafenib ausgewählt [11]. Bislang hat sich der in der SHARP-Studie gezeigte Überlebensvorteil und die Verzögerung zur Progression unter Sorafenib bestätigt – und dies insbesondere für Patienten mit gut erhaltener Leberfunktion (Child-Pugh A). Weiterhin ist unklar, ob die Therapie mit Sorafenib auch zu einem Überlebensvorteil bei Patienten im Stadium Child-Pugh B führt. Entsprechend wird in der aktuellen S3-Leitlinie die Empfehlung zur Therapie mit Sorafenib primär für Patienten mit Child-Pugh A ausgesprochen. Bei Patienten im frühen Stadium von Child-Pugh B (7 Punkte) muss eine individuelle Therapieentscheidung getroffen werden.

Sunitinib

Nach der erfolgreichen Phase-III-Studie mit Sorafenib wurde eine Reihe weiterer antiangiogenetisch wirksamer Substanzen für die Therapie des HCC sowohl bei therapienaiven Patienten als auch bei Patienten nach Sorafenib-Versagen oder -Unverträglichkeit untersucht (Tab. 1).

Erste Erfolg versprechende Ergebnisse aus Phase-II-Studien lieferten die Grundlage für eine Phase-III-Vergleichsstudie mit dem antiangiogenetisch und antiproliferativ wirksamen Multikinase-Inhibitor Sunitinib (SUN1170-HCC-Studie) [12, 13], in deren beiden Arme 1073 Patienten – im Gegensatz zur SHARP-Studie auch aus dem asiatischen Raum stammend – randomisiert aufgenommen wurden (544 mit Sorafenib, 529 mit Sunitinib; 24% nichtasiatische Patienten). Das primäre Ziel der Studie war es, die Überlegenheit oder Nichtunterlegenheit von Sunitinib bezüglich der Gesamtüberlebenszeit gegenüber Sorafenib nachzuweisen. Dieses Ziel wurde jedoch nicht erreicht, da die Studie 2010 vorzeitig abgebrochen wurde, nachdem das unabhängige Daten-Monitoring-Komitee (DMC) eine ungünstige Risiko-Nutzen-

Tab. 1. Alternative, getestete antiangiogenetische Inhibitoren im HCC (nach [41–43])

	VEGFR	PDGFR	FGFR	VEGF	c-KIT
Sorafenib	2, 3	√			√
Sunitinib	1, 2	√			√
Axitinib	1, 2, 3				
Brivanib	1, 2, 3		1, 2, 3		
Linifanib	1, 2, 3				√
BIBF 1120	1, 2, 3	√	1, 2, 3		
Bevacizumab				√	
Ramucirumab	2				

Bewertung für die Sunitinib-Gruppe vorgenommen hatte. In dieser waren die Frequenz und der Schweregrad der Nebenwirkungen so hoch, dass dort bei einem vorher geplanten Sicherheitsreview 18% behandlungsbedingte Todesfälle festgestellt wurden. Die anschließende Analyse ergab ein medianes Gesamtüberleben von 7,9 Monaten in der Sunitinib- und von 10,2 Monaten in der Sorafenib-Gruppe (HR 1,30; 95%-KI 1,13–1,50; p = 0,0010) und bestätigte somit die nur auf der SHARP-Studie basierenden Zulassungsdaten für Sorafenib.

In der Subgruppe der nichtasiatischen Patienten mit chronischer Hepatitis C bestätigte sich interessanterweise die besondere Wirksamkeit von Sorafenib in dieser Patientengruppe – mit einer mittleren Überlebenszeit in der Sorafenib-Gruppe von sogar 18,3 Monaten gegenüber 8,6 Monaten in der Sunitinib-Gruppe (HR 1,76; 95%-KI 0,99–3,10; p = 0,0544) (Abb. 4).

Brivanib

Eine weitere interessante antiangiogenetisch wirksame Substanz, die sich derzeit in klinischer Testung befindet, ist Brivanib. Brivanib ist ein oral verfügbarer, selektiver, dualer

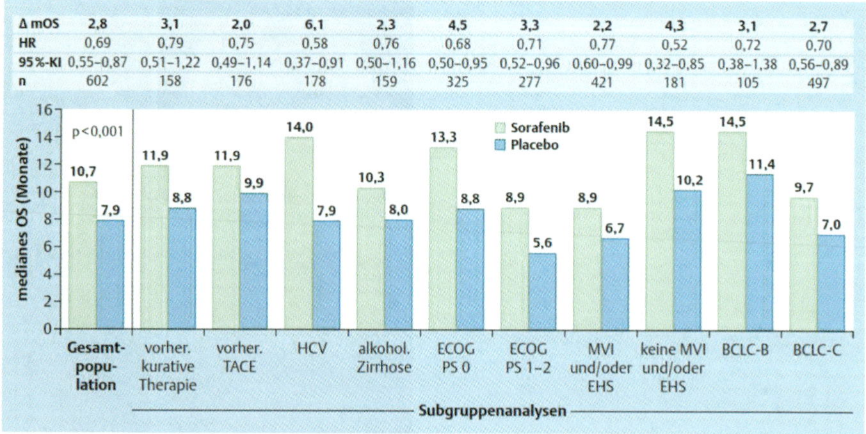

Abb. 4. SHARP-Subgruppenanalyse: Gesamtüberleben (KI = Konfidenzintervall, TACE = transarterielle Chemoembolisation, HCV = Hepatitis-C-Virus, MVI = mikrovaskuläre Invasion, EHS = extrahepatische Ausweitung) (aus [38], mit freundlicher Genehmigung des Georg Thieme Verlags, Stuttgart; modifiziert nach [6–9, 40]).

Inhibitor der VEGF(vaskulärer endothelialer Wachstumsfaktor)- und FGF(Fibroblasten-Wachstumsfaktor)-Rezeptoren, der das Tumorwachstum direkt und indirekt beeinflusst [14–17]. In präklinischen Studien konnten die antitumorösen Eigenschaften von Brivanib in multiplen Tumoren einschließlich des HCC in Sorafenib-resistenten Tumormodellen gezeigt werden [14, 18, 19]. Diese präklinischen Ergebnisse wurden auf die Induktion von FGF bei Sorafenib-resistenten Patienten zurückgeführt und lieferten die Grundlage für eine offene Phase-II-Studie, in der Brivanib (800 mg täglich) zum einen als Second-line-Therapie nach gescheiterter antiangiogenetischer Behandlung [20] und zum anderen als First-line-Therapie bei Patienten mit fortgeschrittenem HCC getestet wurde [21]. Als primäre Endpunkte wurden unter anderem das progressionsfreie Überleben und das Gesamtüberleben vereinbart. In beiden Kohorten konnte bei 40–58% zumindest eine Stabilisierung (stable disease) der Erkrankung erreicht werden. Das mediane Gesamtüberleben war 9,8 Monate (95%-KI 5,5–13,2) in der Second-line- bzw. 10 Monate (95%-KI 6,8–15,2) in der First-line-Kohorte. Die häufigsten Nebenwirkungen waren Fatigue, Appetitlosigkeit, Übelkeit, Diarrhö und Hypertension. Insgesamt zeigte Brivanib ein günstiges Sicherheitsprofil.

Basierend auf diesen Ergebnissen wurden zwei große Phase-III-Erstlinien- und -Zweitlinien-Studien beim HCC initiiert. In der doppelblinden, multizentrischen BRISK-PS-Studie wurde die Wirksamkeit von Brivanib gegenüber Best Supportive Care bei Patienten mit fortgeschrittenem HCC nach Versagen von oder Intoleranz gegenüber Sorafenib untersucht (ClinicalTrials.gov-Identifier: NCT00825955). In dieser Studie wurden 395 Patienten aus Europa (42%), Asien (41%) und Amerika (17%) eingeschlossen. Die große Mehrheit (85%) bestand aus Männern mit einem medianen Alter knapp über 60 Jahren. Stratifiziert wurde nach Intoleranz gegenüber oder Progress unter Sorafenib, nach ECOG-Performance-Status 0 versus 1–2 und dem Vorhandensein oder Fehlen von makroskopischer Gefäßinvasion und/oder extrahepatischen Metastasen. Ende 2011 zeigte sich allerdings, dass das Gesamtüberleben unter Brivanib im Vergleich zu Placebo nicht signifikant verbessert werden konnte. Überraschenderweise hatten insbesondere Patienten mit großem Tumor (10 cm), hohem Alpha-Fetoprotein, extrahepatischer Manifestation und/oder makroskopischer Gefäßinvasion nicht von der Behandlung mit Brivanib profitiert.

In der zweiten Phase-III-Studie wurde Brivanib gegenüber Sorafenib als First-line-Behandlung bei Patienten mit fortgeschrittenem HCC (BRISK-FL-Studie) untersucht (ClinicalTrials.gov-Identifier: NCT00858871). 1050 Patienten mit fortgeschrittenem HCC ohne vorherige systemische Behandlung wurden in der randomisierten, doppelblinden, multizentrischen Phase-III-Studie eingeschlossen. Allerdings wurde auch hier der primäre Endpunkt, also eine Nichtunterlegenheit von Brivanib gegenüber Sorafenib, bei diesem gut ausgewogenen Patientenkollektiv nicht erreicht. Basierend auf diesen sehr enttäuschenden Daten wurden alle Studienprogramme von Brivanib bei HCC eingestellt.

EGFR-Signalweg

Neben den antiangiogenetischen Therapien wurden zunehmend auch andere molekulare Signalwege als mögliche Angriffspunkte für eine systemische Therapie bei Patienten mit fortgeschrittenem HCC untersucht.

In Anbetracht der wichtigen Rolle des EGFR-Signalwegs bei vielen Tumorentitäten und den dort erfolgreich beendeten Studien stellten die entsprechenden molekularen Inhibitoren hierbei eine der als Erstes untersuchten Gruppen dar. Alle bislang publizierten Phase-II- und -III-Studien, die die EGFR-Inhibitoren Erlotinib [22–24], Gefitinib [25], Lapatinib [26] und Cetuximab [27] bei Patienten mit fortgeschrittenem HCC untersuchten, haben bislang allerdings keine überzeugende antitumorale Wirksamkeit nachweisen können.

Erlotinib ist ein selektiver Inhibitor der Tyrosinkinase-Domäne des EGFR, der beim fortgeschrittenen oder metastasierten nichtkleinzelligen Bronchialkarzinom (non-small-cell lung carcinoma, NSCLC) zugelassen ist und auch bereits beim HCC in kleineren Phase-II-Studien getestet wurde [22–24]. Die Ergebnisse dieser Studien ließen vermuten, dass diese Substanz in der Kombination mit Sorafenib eine Aktivität beim HCC hat, und veranlassten die Initiierung der SEARCH-Studie, einer internationalen, multizentrischen, placebokontrollierten Phase-III-Studie, in der 720 Patienten mit fortgeschrittenem HCC randomisiert wurden. Verglichen wurde primär das mittlere Gesamtüberleben unter Sorafenib plus Placebo gegenüber Sorafenib plus Erlotinib. Im Juli 2012 wurde bekannt, dass die Kombination mit Erlotinib kein verbessertes Überleben im Vergleich zu einer alleinigen Therapie mit Sorafenib erbrachte, sodass insgesamt nicht zu erwarten ist, dass Inhibitoren des EGFR-Signalwegs eine Rolle bei der Therapie des HCC spielen werden.

RAF/MEK/ERK-Signalweg

Die molekularen Mechanismen der Wirksamkeit von Sorafenib sind bis heute nicht gut verstanden. Aufgrund seiner Aktivität gegenüber dem RAF-Signalweg, der in 50–60% der HCCs aktiviert ist, entwickelte sich in den vergangenen Jahren ein wachsendes Interesse an diesem RAF/MEK(Mitogen-aktivierte Proteinkinase)/ERK-Signalweg, und der oral verfügbare Inhibitor der MEK-Tyrosinkinase Selumetinib wurde in einer Phase-II-Studie bei Patienten mit fortgeschrittenem HCC ohne vorherige Behandlung getestet [28]. Entgegen der großen Erwartungen konnte in dieser Studie allerdings kein radiologisches Ansprechen verzeichnet und die Zeit zur Progression nicht verlängert werden.

mTOR-Signalweg

«Mammalian target of rapamycin» (mTOR) ist ein zentraler Regulator einer Reihe von zellulären Prozessen, die von hohem onkologischen Interesse sind. In vielen Tumorentitäten, inklusive dem HCC, wurde zudem eine deutliche Aktivierung dieses Signalwegs nachgewiesen und korreliert beim HCC z.B. mit dem Risiko eines Rezidivs nach Resektion [29]. Präklinische Studien haben zudem gezeigt, dass mTOR-Inhibitoren effektiv das Zellwachstum und die Gefäßinvasion in HCC-Zelllinien in vitro und in HCC-Tumormodellen in vivo hemmen [29–31]. Verschiedene mTOR-Inhibitoren (Sirolimus, Temsirolimus und Everolimus) sind derzeit in klinischer Erprobung beim HCC. In der SilVER05-Studie wird untersucht, ob durch Sirolimus im Vergleich zu einer mTOR-Inhibitor-freien Immunsuppression das Risiko eines HCC-Rezidivs nach Lebertransplantation verringert werden kann. In diese Studie konnten alle geplanten Patienten eingeschlossen werden; diese befinden sich derzeit in der Nachbeobachtungsphase (Sirolimus-containing versus mTOR-inhibitor-free immunosuppression in patients undergoing liver transplantation for hepatocellular carcinoma; ClinicalTrials.gov-Identifier: NCT00355862). In der palliativen Situation wurde in einer großen Phase-III-Studie die Wirksamkeit von Everolimus bei Patienten mit Sorafenib-Versagen/Unverträglichkeit bei über 700 Patienten untersucht (Evolve-1-Studie, ClinicalTrials.gov-Identifier: NCT00345839). Diese Studie wurde nicht vorzeitig beendet; die Ergebnisse werden für 2013 erwartet.

Tab. 2. Ergebnisse der randomisierten Phase-II-Studie mit Tivantinib (nach [37])

	Tivantinib	Placebo	HR (KI[a])	p-Wert
Median TTP, Wochen				
ITT	6,9	6,0	0,64 (0,43–0,94)	0,04
MET[hoch]	11,7	6,1	0,43 (0,19–0,97)	0,03
Median OS, Monate				
ITT	6,6	6,2	0,90 (0,57–1,40)	0,63
MET[hoch]	7,2	3,8	0,38 (0,18–0,81)	0,01

[a]90%-KI für primäre TTP; 95%-KI für andere Endpunkte.
TTP = Mittlere Tumorprogressionszeit; ITT = Intent-to-Treat-Population; OS = Gesamtüberleben.

C-MET/HGF-Signalweg

Eine Substanzgruppe von derzeit sehr hohem Interesse bei einer Vielzahl von Tumorentitäten sind Inhibitoren der Rezeptor-Tyrosinkinase c-MET mit seinem Liganden, dem Hepatozyten-Wachstumsfaktor (hepatocyte growth factor, HGF). C-MET spielt eine wichtige Rolle im Zell- und Tumorwachstum, und eine Überexpression/Aktivierung von c-MET konnte beim HCC in einer Reihe von retrospektiven Analysen gezeigt werden [32–35]. Cabozantinib (XL184) ist ein oral verfügbarer, dualer MET/VEGFR2-Inhibitor. Dieser wurde gegenüber Placebo in einer Phase-II-Diskontinuitätsstudie bei 41 Child-Pugh-A-Patienten mit progredientem HCC und maximal einer einzigen Vorbehandlung entweder als First- oder Second-line-Behandlung untersucht [36]. Als primäre Endpunkte wurden die Gesamt-Ansprechrate nach mRECIST und das progressionsfreie Überleben festgelegt. Mit einem progressionsfreien Überleben von 4,4 Monaten und einem medianen Gesamtüberleben von 15,1 Monaten zeigte Cabozantinib eine beachtliche antitumorale Wirkung bei Patienten mit fortgeschrittenem HCC.

Ein weiterer Erfolg versprechender c-MET-Inhibitor ist Tivantinib (ARQ197), ein selektiver, non-ATP-kompetitiver Inhibitor der MET-Tyrosinkinase. Tivantinib wurde kürzlich in einer multizentrischen, placebokontrollierten, doppelblinden Phase-II-Studie untersucht [37]. 107 Patienten mit fortgeschrittenem HCC und Child-Pugh-A-Zirrhose, die unter First-line-Therapie progredient oder dieser gegenüber intolerant waren, wurden in die Studie eingeschlossen. Primärer Endpunkt dieser Studie war die Zeit bis zur radiologisch gesicherten Progression. Erfreulicherweise wurde schon vorab festgelegt, Tumorgewebe zentral zu asservieren und zwecks Beurteilung der c-MET-Expression immunhistochemisch aufzuarbeiten. In der gesamten Population konnte keine Verbesserung des Überlebens durch die Therapie mit Tivantinib erreicht werden. Interessanterweise konnte in dieser Studie allerdings c-MET prospektiv als negativer prognostischer Faktor identifiziert werden; d.h., Patienten mit einer Überexpression von c-MET wiesen ein signifikant kürzeres Überleben auf als jene ohne C-MET-Expression. Durch die Therapie mit Tivantinib bei c-MET-überexprimierenden Patienten konnte eine signifikante Verlängerung des Gesamtüberlebens von 7,2 Monaten im Vergleich zu 3,8 Monaten in der Placebo-Gruppe sowie eine signifikante Verlängerung der Zeit zur Progression erreicht werden (Tab. 2). Basierend auf diesen positiven Daten wird in Kürze eine Phase-III-Studie zur Evaluierung von Tivantinib als Second-line-Behandlung bei c-MET-überexprimierenden Patienten begonnen.

Schlussfolgerungen

Das HCC ist eine der häufigsten Tumorerkrankungen und tumorvermittelten Todesursachen weltweit. Mit dem Multikinase-Inhibitor Sorafenib konnte erstmals ein signifikanter Überlebensvorteil bei Patienten mit fortgeschrittenem HCC gezeigt werden. Bis heute ist Sorafenib die einzige zugelassene systemisch wirksame Substanz für Patienten mit fortgeschrittenem HCC. Die Behandlungsoptionen sind jedoch beschränkt. Es fehlen Second-line-Therapien für Patienten, die Sorafenib nicht tolerieren und/oder hierunter progredient werden.

Neue molekulare Therapien befinden sich in klinischer Entwicklung, bislang allerdings mit zumeist negativen Ergebnissen. Die getesteten alternativen Angiogenese-Inhibitoren Sunitinib und Brivanib konnten in Phase-III-Studien keine Verlängerung des Gesamtüberlebens zeigen. Eine andere, initial vielversprechende Zielgruppe stellten die EGFR-Inhibitoren dar. Leider erwiesen sich auch diese weder als Alternative zu noch als Option zur Kombination mit Sorafenib. Andere interessante molekulare Substanzen wie Inhibitoren von mTOR, PI3K/Akt und IGFR befinden sich in teils noch früher klinischer Entwicklung.

Aktuell Erfolg versprechend erscheint die Inhibition von c-MET. Eine Phase-II-Studie mit dem c-MET-Inhibitor Tivantinib zeigte erstmals bei c-MET-überexprimierenden Patienten eine signifikante Verlängerung des Überlebens sowie der Zeit zur Progression. Die Entwicklung der systemischen Behandlung des HCC bleibt anspruchsvoll. Zunehmend wird jedoch ersichtlich, dass die große Herausforderung in der Identifikation von prognostischen und prädiktiven Faktoren für eine personalisierte Therapie besteht.

Disclosure Statement

Die Verfasser haben keinen Interessenkonflikt zu offenbaren.

Literatur

1 El-Serag HB: Hepatocellular carcinoma. N Engl J Med 2011;365:1118–1127.

2 European Association for the Study of the Liver; European Organisation for Research and Treatment of Cancer: EASL-EORTC clinical practical guidelines: management of hepatocellular carcinoma. J Hepatol 2012;56:908–943.

3 Bruix J, Sherman M: Management of hepatocellular carcinoma: an update. Hepatology 2011;53: 1020–1022.

4 Abou-Alfa GK, Schwartz L, Ricci S, Amadori D, Santoro A, Figer A, De Greve J, Douillard JY, Lathia C, Schwartz B, Taylor I, Moscovici M, Saltz LB: Phase II study of sorafenib in patients with advanced hepatocellular carcinoma. J Clin Oncol 2006;24:4293–4300.

5 Llovet JM, Ricci S, Mazzaferro V, et al.; SHARP Investigators Study Group: Sorafenib in advanced hepatocellular carcinoma. N Engl J Med 2008;359: 378–390.

6 Galle P, Blanc J, Van Laethem J-L, Marrero J, Beaugrand M, Moscovici M, Shan M, Nadel A, Voliotis D, Bruix J, Lovet JM: Efficacy and safety of sorafenib in patients with advanced hepatocellular carcinoma and prior anti-tumor therapy: a subanalysis from the sharp trial. J Hepatol 2008;48 (suppl 2):S372.

7 Bolondi L, Caspary W, Bennouna J, Thomson B, Van Steenbergen W, Degos F, Shan M, Moscovici M, Llovet J, Bruix J: Clinical benefit of sorafenib in hepatitis C patients with hepatocellular carcinoma (HCC): subgroup analysis of the SHARP trial. Gastrointestinal Cancers Symposium 2008;abstr 129.

8 Craxi A, Porta C, Sangiovanni A, Seitz J, Moscovici M, Shan M, Nadel A, Voliotis D, Bruix J, Llovet JM: Efficacy and safety of sorafenib in patients with alcohol-related hepatocellular carcinoma: a sub-analysis from the SHARP trial. J Clin Oncol 2008;26(suppl):abstr 15591.

9 Bruix J, Cheng A, Kang Y , Tsao C, Qin S, Lentini G, Zou J, Nadel A, Burock K, Voliotis D, Llovet JM: Effect of macroscopic vascular invasion (MVI), extrahepatic spread (EHS), and ECOG performance status (ECOG PS) on outcome in patients with advanced hepatocellular carcinoma (HCC) treated with sorafenib: analysis of two phase III, randomized, double-blind trials. J Clin Oncol 2009;27(suppl 15):abstr 4580.

10 Ren Z, Zhu K, Kang H, Lu M, Qu Z, Lu L, Song T, Zhou W, Wang H, Yang W, Wang X, Yang Y, Shi L, Bai Y, Ye S-L: A randomized controlled phase II study of the prophylactic effect of urea-based cream on the hand-foot skin reaction associated with sorafenib in advanced hepatocellular carcinoma. ASCO Annual Meeting 2012;abstr 4008.

11 Lencioni R, Marrero J, Venook A, Ye SL, Kudo M: Design and rationale for the non-interventional Global Investigation of therapeutic DEcisions in hepatocellular carcinoma and Of its treatment with sorafeNib (GIDEON) study. Int J Clin Pract 2010; 64:1034–1041.

12 Faivre S, Raymond E, Boucher E, Douillard J, Lim HY, Kim JS, Zappa M, Lanzalone S, Lin X, Deprimo S, Harmon C, Ruiz-Garcia A, Lechuga MJ, Cheng AL: Safety and efficacy of sunitinib in patients with advanced hepatocellular carcinoma: an open-label, multicentre, phase II study. Lancet Oncol 2009;10:794–800.

13 Cheng A, Kang Y, Lin D, Park J, Kudo M, Qin S, Omata M, Pitman Lowenthal SW, Lanzalone S, Yang L, Lechuga M, Raymond E: Phase III trial of sunitinib (Su) versus sorafenib (So) in advanced hepatocellular carcinoma (HCC). J Clin Oncol 2011;29(suppl):abstr 4000.

14 Bhide RS, Lombardo LJ, Hunt JT, Cai ZW, Barrish JC, Galbraith S, Jeyaseelan R Sr, Mortillo S, Wautlet BS, Krishnan B, Kukral D, Malone H, Lewin AC, Henley BJ, Fargnoli J: The antiangiogenic activity in xenograft models of brivanib, a dual inhibitor of vascular endothelial growth factor receptor-2 and fibroblast growth factor receptor-1 kinases. Mol Cancer Ther 2010;9:369–370.

15 Dailey L, Ambrosetti D, Mansukhani A, Basilico C: Mechanisms underlying differential responses to FGF signaling. Cytokine Growth Factor Rev 2005; 16:233–247.

16 Korc M, Friesel RE: The role of fibroblast growth factors in tumor growth. Curr Cancer Drug Targets 2009;9:630–651.

17 Saylor PJ, Escudier B, Michaelson MD: Importance of fibroblast growth factor receptor in neovascularization and tumor escape from antiangiogenic therapy. Clin Genitourin Cancer 2012;10:77–83.

18 Huynh H, Ngo VC, Fargnol J, Ayers M, Soo KC, Koong HN, Thng CH, Ong HS, Chung A, Chow P, Pollock P, Byron S, Tran E: Brivanib alaninate, a dual inhibitor of vascular endothelial growth factor receptor and fibroblast growth factor receptor tyrosine kinases, induces growth inhibition in mouse models of human hepatocellular carcinoma. Clin Cancer Res 2006;14:6145–6153.

19 Tovar V: FGF signaling dysregulation in HCC and role in the development of acquired resistance to anti-angiogenic therapies. HCA 2011;abstr 0–006.

20 Finn RS, Kang YK, Mulcahy M, Polite BN, Lim HY, Walters I, Baudelet C, Manekas D, Park JW: Phase II, open-label study of brivanib as second-line therapy in patients with advanced hepatocellular carcinoma. Clin Cancer Res 2012;18:1–9.
21 Park JW, Finn RS, Kim JS, Karwal M, Li RK, Ismail F, Thomas M, Harris R, Baudelet C, Walters I, Raoul JL: Phase II, open-label study of brivanib as first-line therapy in patients with advanced hepatocellular carcinoma. Clin Cancer Res 2011;17:1973–1983.
22 Philip PA, Mahoney MR, Allmer C, et al: Phase II study of Erlotinib (OSI-774) in patients with advanced hepatocellular cancer. J Clin Oncol 2005;23:6657–6663.
23 Thomas MB, Chadha R, Glover K, Chadha R, Iwasaki M, Kaur H, Lin E, Kaseb A, Glover K, Davila M, Abbruzzese J: Phase 2 study of erlotinib in patients with unresectable hepatocellular carcinoma. Cancer 2007;110:1059–1067.
24 Thomas MB, Morris JS, Chadha R, Iwasaki M, Kaur H, Lin E, Kaseb A, Glover K, Davila M, Abbruzzese J: Phase II trial of the combination of bevacizumab and erlotinib in patients who have advanced hepatocellular carcinoma. J Clin Oncol 2009;27:843–850.
25 O'Dwyer PJ, Giantonio BJ, Levy DE, Kauh JS, Fitzgerald DB, Benson AB: Gefitinib in advanced unresectable hepatocellular carcinoma: results from the Eastern Cooperative Oncology Group's Study E1203. J Clin Oncol 2006;24(suppl):4143.
26 Ramanathan RK, Belani CP, Singh DA, Tanaka M, Lenz HJ, Yen Y, Kindler HL, Iqbal S, Longmate J, Mack PC, Lurje G, Gandour-Edwards R, Dancey J, Gandara DR: A phase II study of lapatinib in patients with advanced biliary tree and hepatocellular cancer. Cancer Chemother Pharmacol 2009;64:777–783.
27 Zhu AX, Stuart K, Blaszkowsky LS, Muzikansky A, Reitberg DP, Clark JW, Enzinger PC, Bhargava P, Meyerhardt JA, Horgan K, Fuchs CS, Ryan DP: Phase 2 study of cetuximab in patients with advanced hepatocellular carcinoma. Cancer 2007;110:581–589.
28 O'Neil BH, Goff LW, Kauh JS, Strosberg JR, Bekaii-Saab TS, Lee RM, Kazi A, Moore DT, Learoyd M, Lush RM, Sebti SM, Sullivan DM: Phase II study of the mitogen-activated protein kinase 1/2 inhibitor selumetinib in patients with advanced hepatocellular carcinoma. J Clin Oncol 2011;29:2350–2356.
29 Villanueva A, Chiang DY, Newell P, et al: Pivotal role of mTOR signaling in hepatocellular carcinoma. Gastroenterology 2008;135:1972–1983, 1983.e1–11.
30 Sahin F, Kannangai R, Adegbola O, Wang J, Su G, Torbenson M: mTOR and P70 S6 kinase expression in primary liver neoplasms. Clin Cancer Res 2004;10:8421–8425.
31 Buitrago-Molina LE, Pothiraju D, Lamle J, et al: Rapamycin delays tumor development in murine livers by inhibiting proliferation of hepatocytes with DNA damage. Hepatology 2009;50:500–509.
32 Birchmeier C, Birchmeier W, Gherardi E, Vande Woude GF: Met, metastasis, motility and more. Nat Rev Mol Cell Biol 2003;4:915–925.
33 Ueki T, Fujimoto J, Suzuki T, Yamamoto H, Okamoto E: Expression of hepatocyte growth factor and its receptor, the c-met proto-oncogene, in hepatocellular carcinoma. Hepatology 1997;25:619–623.
34 Kaposi-Novak P, Lee JS, Gomez-Quiroz L, Coulouarn C, Factor VM, Thorgeirsson SS: Met-regulated expression signature defines a subset of human hepatocellular carcinomas with poor prognosis and aggressive phenotype. J Clin Invest 2006;116:1582–1595.
35 Ke AW, Shi GM, Zhou J, Wu FZ, Ding ZB, Hu MY, Xu Y, Song ZJ, Wang ZJ, Wu JC, Bai DS, Li JC, Liu KD, Fan J: Role of overexpression of CD151 and/or c-Met in predicting prognosis of hepatocellular carcinoma. Hepatology 2009;49:491–503.
36 Cohn AL, Kelley RK, Yang T-S, Su W-C, Verslype C, Ramies DA, Lee Y, Shen X, Van Cutsem E: Activity of cabozantinib (XL184) in hepatocellular carcinoma patients (pts): results from a phase II randomized discontinuation trial (RDT). J Clin Oncol 2012;30(suppl 4):abstr 261.
37 Santoro A, Rimassa L, Borbath I, et al: Tivantinib for second-line treatment of advanced hepatocellular carcinoma: a randomised, placebo-controlled phase 2 study. Lancet Oncol 2013;14:55–63.
38 Ganten T, et al: Fortschritte in der Behandlung des hepatozellulären Karzinoms. Thieme-Refresher Innere Medizin 2012;R1–R16.
39 Lipworth AD, Robert C, Zhu AX: Hand-foot syndrome (hand-foot skin reaction, palmar-plantar erythrodysesthesia): focus on sorafenib and sunitinib. Oncology 2009;77:257–271.
40 Bruix J, Raoul JL, Sherman M, Shan M, Lentini G, Nadel A, Voliotis D, Llovet JM: Efficacy and safety of sorafenib in patients with hepatocellular carcinoma (HCC): subanalysis of SHARP trial based on Barcelona Clinic Liver Cancer (BCLC) stage. J Hepatol 2009;50(suppl 1):S28–S29.
41 Finn R: Development of molecularly targeted therapies in hepatocellular carcinoma: where do we go now? Clin Cancer Res 2010;16:390–397.
42 Kelly RJ, Rixe O: Axitinib – a selective inhibitor of the vascular endothelial growth factor (VEGF) receptor. Target Oncol 2009;4:297–305.
43 Villanueva A, Llovet JM: Targeted therapies for hepatocellular carcinoma. Gastroenterology 2011;140:1410–1426.

Viszeralmedizin
Gastrointestinal Medicine and Surgery

Review Article · Übersichtsarbeit

Viszeralmedizin 2013;29:92–102
DOI: 10.1159/000350732

Online publiziert: 15. April 2013

Locoregional Transarterial Therapies for Hepatocellular Carcinoma: Transarterial Chemoembolization and Radioembolization

Mercedes Iñarrairaegui[a,b] Delia D'Avola[a,b] Bruno Sangro[a,b]

[a] Liver Unit, Clinica Universidad de Navarra, Pamplona,
[b] Centro de Investigacion Biomedica en Red de Enfermedades Hepaticas y Digestivas (CIBERehd), Barcelona, Spain

Keywords
Hepatocellular carcinoma, HCC · Chemoembolization · Radioembolization

Summary
Background: Hepatocellular carcinoma (HCC) is the sixth most common cancer in the world and the third most common cause of cancer-related mortality. Despite the widespread implementation of surveillance programs, more than half of the patients with HCC are diagnosed at late stages, when curative treatments (resection or liver transplantation) cannot be applied. For patients presenting with unresectable, non-transplantable HCC and a relatively preserved liver function, locoregional transarterial therapies are the main therapeutic options. Therefore, locoregional transarterial treatments play a key role in the management of HCC. The concept of catheter transarterial therapies is to selectively deliver anticancer treatments to liver tumors. This is possible due to the unique double irrigation of the liver and the predominantly arterial irrigation of liver tumors. **Method:** An exhaustive analysis of the literature, focused mainly on the last 25 years, has been carried out. **Results:** This review discusses the scientific evidence supporting the use of transarterial therapies for patients with HCC, including chemoembolization with conventional materials or drug-eluting beads, and internal radiation procedures such as the injection of radiation-loaded microspheres. **Conclusion:** Transarterial chemoembolization has been shown to improve the survival of those patients with unresectable HCC who have a preserved liver function and a low tumor burden. Recently developed devices and procedures, particularly drug-eluting beads and radioactive microspheres, may further improve the clinical outcome of patients receiving transarterial therapies. The combination with antiangiogenic agents is an appealing approach that should be explored.

Schlüsselwörter
Hepatozelluläres Karzinom, HCC · Chemoembolisation · Radioembolisation

Zusammenfassung
Hintergrund: Das Leberzellkarzinom (HCC) ist weltweit die sechsthäufigste Krebsart und die dritthäufigste Ursache von krebsbedingter Mortalität. Trotz der weit verbreiteten Anwendung von Überwachungsprogrammen befindet sich mehr als die Hälfte der Patienten mit HCC bei Diagnose bereits in einem späten Stadium, wenn kurative Behandlungen (Resektion oder Lebertransplantation) nicht angewendet werden können. Für Patienten mit inoperablem, nicht transplantierbarem HCC und relativ gut erhaltener Leberfunktion stellen lokoregionäre transarterielle Therapien die wichtigsten therapeutischen Optionen dar. Daher spielen lokoregionale transarterielle Behandlungen eine wichtige Rolle in der Handhabung des HCC. Das Konzept der transarteriellen Kathetertherapien besteht darin, Lebertumoren selektiv mit Anti-Krebs-Therapien zu behandeln. Dies ist aufgrund der einzigartigen doppelten Irrigation der Leber sowie der überwiegend arteriellen Irrigation von Lebertumoren möglich. **Methode:** Eine ausführliche Analyse der Literatur, die sich vor allem auf die letzten 25 Jahre konzentrierte, wurde durchgeführt. **Ergebnisse:** Diese Übersicht diskutiert die wissenschaftlichen Nachweise zur Verwendung von transarteriellen Therapien bei Patienten mit HCC, einschließlich Chemoembolisation mit konventionellen Materialien oder «drug-eluting beads», und internen Radiotherapien wie die Injektion von radioaktiven Mikrosphären. **Schlussfolgerung:** Für die transarterielle Chemoembolisation konnte gezeigt werden, dass das Überleben von Patienten mit inoperablem HCC, die eine erhaltene Leberfunktion und eine geringe Tumorlast aufweisen, verbessert wurde. Kürzlich entwickelte Geräte und Verfahren, insbesondere «drug-eluting beads» und radioaktive Mikrosphären, könnten das klinische Outcome der Patienten, die transarterielle Therapien erhalten, weiter verbessern. Die Kombination mit antiangiogenen Substanzen ist ein vielversprechender Ansatz, dem weiter nachgegangen werden sollte.

KARGER
Fax +49 761 4 52 07 14
Information@Karger.com
www.karger.com

1662-6664/13/0292-0092$38.00/0

Accessible online at:
www.karger.com/vim

Mercedes Iñarrairaegui, MD, PhD
Liver Unit, Clinica Universidad de Navarra
Avenida Pio XII 36, 31008 Pamplona, Spain
minarra@unav.es

Introduction

Hepatocellular carcinoma (HCC) is the sixth most common cancer in the world and the third most common cause of cancer-related mortality [1]. Cirrhotic patients are at a special risk of developing HCC, and this underlying liver disease impacts both on the therapeutic decision and the survival [2]. Early diagnosis of HCC can be achieved by surveillance of at-risk populations [3, 4]. Despite the widespread implementation of surveillance programs, more than half of the patients with HCC are diagnosed at late stages when curative treatments (resection or liver transplantation) cannot be applied [5]. For patients presenting with unresectable, non-transplantable HCC and a relatively preserved liver function, locoregional transarterial therapies are the main therapeutic options.

Locoregional transarterial therapies for unresectable HCC consist of a catheter-based group of treatments where therapeutic and/or embolic agents are intra-arterially directed to target tumors. The unique double irrigation of the liver and the predominantly arterial irrigation of liver tumors, particularly primary liver cancer, are at the core of all transarterial therapies. The most common techniques used in HCC treatment are transarterial chemoembolization (TACE) with or without drug-eluting beads (DEB) and Yttrium 90 (90Y) radioembolization (90Y-RE). TACE combines local and targeted drug delivery with concurrent tumor-feeding artery embolization. 90Y-RE is a form of brachytherapy in which intra-arterially injected microspheres loaded with 90Y serve as sources for internal radiation purposes.

This review focuses on these transarterial procedures and their role in the management of patients with HCC. It has to be stressed that the scientific evidence supporting the use of locoregional transarterial therapy is heterogeneous. The results of clinical trials aimed at investigating the benefit of transarterial therapies in different groups of patients as well as the synergies between locoregional and systemic therapies will be available in the coming years.

Transarterial Chemoembolization

TACE comprises a wide variety of procedures that share two different aims: i) to increase the exposure of tumor cells to chemotherapeutic agents; and ii) to induce ischemic necrosis. To achieve these two goals, TACE procedures involve the injection of chemotherapeutic agents usually followed by the injection of embolizing particles.

Several variations of this technique have been demonstrated throughout the world and no standard protocol has been uniformly adopted. Centers have differed in the choice and/or dose of the anticancer agents used, anticancer agent alone or mixed with lipiodol, the choice of the embolizing agent used, selectivity of catheter positioning, embolization endpoints, and the schedule and/or interval of retreatment [6]. This heterogeneity makes the analysis of the literature even more complicated.

Although conventional TACE with administration of an anticancer-in-lipiodol emulsion followed by embolic agents has been the most popular technique, bland embolization is still preferred in some centers, and TACE with drug-eluting particles (DEB-TACE) has replaced conventional regimens in others.

Conventional Tace

Technical Considerations

TACE is currently defined as the infusion of a mixture of chemotherapeutic agents with or without iodized oil, followed by an embolization with particles. In treating HCC, single-agent doxorubicin is commonly used, whereas the combination of mitomycin C, doxorubicin, and cisplatin is preferred in the United States. Irrespective of the agent used, it is typically emulsified in lipiodol, an oily contrast agent believed to increase intratumoral retention of the cytotoxic agent. Iodized oil has been shown to act as a carrier of chemotherapeutic agents which are slowly released from the lipiodol mixture [7, 8]. The iodized oil persists selectively in the tumor for a few weeks or months because of hemodynamic differences between hypervascular hepatic tumors and liver parenchyma and presumably because of the absence of Kupffer cells in tumors [9]. This is followed by embolization of the target vessels with agents such as gelfoam (heterogeneous in size), the more recently calibrated polyvinyl alcohol, or acrylic copolymer gelatin particles [10]. The use of calibrated particles is increasing worldwide as they can be selected by size according to the vessel that needs to be blocked [11]. Vessel occlusion after injection of the chemotherapeutic mixture results in lower peak plasma concentration and increased drug retention inside the tumors [8]. Induced ischemic necrosis might result in the failure of transmembrane pumps in tumor cells, allowing a greater absorption of chemotherapeutic agents by the tumor [12].

However, the therapeutic benefit obtained from adding a chemotherapeutic agent or lipiodol to bland embolization was challenged by the results of two clinical trials conducted in the 1990s [13, 14]. Furthermore, two meta-analyses found similar outcomes after TACE or bland embolization [6, 15], suggesting that the antitumoral effect is mainly ischemic in nature. Nevertheless, in the following sections we will discuss only TACE as it is the most widely used transarterial embolizing procedure for HCC.

Clinical Evidence

The clinical evidence that supports the use of TACE for the palliative treatment of unresectable HCC comes from the positive results of two randomized controlled trials [16, 17] in

Table 1. Median survival after 90Y-RE and TACE (conventional and DEB-TACE) according to tumor stage (BCLC)

BCLC	Author, year [reference]	N	Median survival, months (95% CI)		
			90Y-RE	cTACE	TACE-DCBeads
A	Salem et al., 2010 [83]	48	26.9 (17.0–30.2)	–	–
	Sangro et al., 2011 [85]	52	24.4 (18.6–38.1)	–	–
	Salem et al., 2011 [35]	43/47	27.3 (17.1–30.2)	45.4 (15.1–46.1)	–
	Wang et al., 2008 [36]	453	–	35.4	–
	Ho et al., 2009 [33]	80	–	29.9	–
	Chen et al., 2009 [31]	n.r.	–	16.8	–
	Lewandowski et al., 2010 [34]	62	–	40 (15–46)	–
	Hsu et al., 2011 [32]	73	–	37.9	–
	Burrel et al., 2012 [63]	41	–	–	40.6 (12.8–84.4)
B	Salem et al., 2010 [83]	83	17.2 (13.5–29.6)	–	–
	Hilgard et al., 2010 [84]	51	16.4 (12.1–∞)	–	–
	Sangro et al., 2011 [85]	87	16.9 (12.8–22.8)	–	–
	Mazzaferro et al., 2013 [86]	17	18 (12–38)	–	–
	Salem et al., 2011 [36]	53/50	17.2 (11.4–29.6)	17.2 (14.8–18.7)	–
	Wang et al., 2008 [37]	741	–	18.2	–
	Chen et al., 2009 [31]	n.r.	–	15.6	–
	Ho et al., 2009 [33]	163	–	16.8	–
	Lewandowski et al., 2010 [34]	73	–	17.4 (13.9–18.8)	–
	Burrel et al., 2012 [63]	63	–	–	42.8 (27.6–58.0)
C	Salem et al., 2010 [83]	107 no EHD	7.3 (6.5–10.1)	–	–
	Salem et al., 2010 [83]	45 EHD	5.4 (2.7–7.5)	–	–
	Sangro et al., 2011 [85]	183	10 (7.7–10.9)	–	–
	Mazzaferro et al., 2013 [86]	35	13 (9.0–17.0)	–	–
	Salem et al., 2011 [36]	13/12 no PI	22.1 (11.2–n.r.)	9.3 (6.2–11.5)	–
	Lewandowski et al., 2010 [34]	23	–	6.6 (4.0–9.3)	–
	Wang et al., 2008 [37]	200	–	6.8	–
	Ho et al., 2009 [33]	48	–	13.6	–
	Chen et al., 2009 [31]	n.r.	–	12.7	–

EHD = Extrahepatic disease; n.r. = not reported; PI = portal invasion.

selected patients with preserved liver function. Llovet et al. [16] prospectively studied the survival outcomes of patients treated with fixed interval (intention to treat) chemoembolization, embolization, and conservative measures. Survival outcomes showed a benefit in highly selected patients (younger than 75 years, free from main portal vein thrombosis (PVT), and preserved liver function) treated with chemoembolization and embolization versus those treated conservatively. The 2-year survival after conventional TACE reached 63% compared to 27% of the untreated control arm ($p = 0.009$). In a second randomized controlled trial, Lo et al. [17] used broader enrollment criteria with the inclusion of patients with limited PVT resulting in a 2-year survival of only 31%, although this outcome was still superior to that of the untreated control group (2-year survival 11%; $p = 0.002$). Three other clinical trials failed to show the superiority of TACE in terms of survival compared to best supportive care or other not effective systemic treatments such as tamoxifen [18–20].

Unlike negative trials, the two trials with positive results recruited patients with slightly lower bilirubin levels, had a higher proportion of patients with one or two tumor nodules, and differed greatly in the etiology of HCC (mainly viral hepatitis in the two positive trials), while alcohol-related chronic liver disease was present in more than 70% of the patients in the negative trials.

However, three meta-analyses [6, 15, 21] have concluded that TACE improves the survival of patients with unresectable HCC. Most patients included in the meta-analysis had a fully preserved liver function (normal median values for total bilirubin, serum albumin, or prothrombin time) and a rather small tumor burden (either single lesions or multiple tumors affecting a single lobe with a median tumor size of 5–7 cm and a small proportion of patients with elevated alpha-fetoprotein (AFP)).

Based on these results, TACE has been established as the standard of care for patients who meet the criteria for the intermediate stage of the Barcelona Clinic Liver Cancer (BCLC) staging system, i.e., those with multinodular HCC, relatively preserved liver function, absence of cancer-related symptoms, and no evidence of vascular invasion or extrahepatic spread [2, 22].

However, in clinical practice, TACE has been applied to patients in other stages than the intermediate one; hence, survival is very heterogeneous and usually worse than that reported in clinical trials, as would be expected in a population that includes more diverse patients regarding liver function and tumor stage. Survival ranges widely in different series from 53 to 90% at 1 year, from 11 to 67% at 2 years, and from 8 to 26% at 5 years, reflecting the heterogeneous population treated [23–31]. According to the BCLC classification (table 1), reported survival ranges from 16 to 45 months in BCLC-A stage, from 15.6 to 18.2 months in BCLC-B stage, and between 6.8 and 13.6 in BCLC-C patients [31–36]. It has to be stressed that similar to other treatments, prognosis after chemoembolization largely depends on liver function [27, 29, 30, 37–39], tumor burden before treatment [23, 29, 30, 40], presence of portal vein invasion [17, 23, 24, 40, 41], and response to treatment [16, 34].

In patients with portal vein invasion, the ischemic effect of TACE has precluded its use because of the risk of inducing liver failure. The extent of PVT that contraindicates TACE is still a matter of debate as patients with involvement of a segmental or lobar branch may achieve long-term outcomes that are much better than those expected from natural history, ranging from 5 to 10 months in some Eastern series with branch thrombosis [42, 43].

Safety Profile

TACE is generally considered a safe procedure. Nevertheless, it is frequently followed by side effects that can eventually be severe. The most common is the postembolization syndrome, consisting of nausea, abdominal pain, and fever. It occurs in more than 40% of patients [44, 45] but is commonly mild and transient. A variable proportion of patients (20–45%) show a transient deterioration of varying degree in liver function after TACE [44, 46], and some series report acute liver decompensation (appearance of ascites, encephalopathy, or jaundice) in 0.1–3% of the cases [18, 45, 47, 48]. In some series, biliary and gastrointestinal tract injury has been reported in 2–10% [49–51] and in 1–5% of the patients [45, 52], respectively. Mortality rates range widely from 0.003 to 10% in the different series [15, 23, 53], reflecting again the heterogeneity in the treatment population as well as the type of regimen and the frequency of the treatment.

Liver functional reserve is a critical component of a careful selection. Patients should present a relatively well-preserved liver function (mostly Child-Pugh A or B7 without ascites), while those with liver decompensation or more advanced liver failure should be excluded since the ischemic insult can lead to severe adverse events. A recent consensus from a panel of experts has recommended a series of absolute and relative contraindications for the treatment of patients at BCLC-B stage, which also applies to the BCLC-C stage since the contraindication for the treatment of PVT is not universally accepted [54].

TACE Using DEB

Technical Considerations

The concept of DEB-TACE is to load embolizing particles with various types of chemotherapeutic agents and to deliver them intra-arterially in a manner similar to that of conventional TACE. These beads are able to take up several drugs by ion exchange in vitro in a fixed dosing and to release them in vivo in a sustained fashion after intra-arterial injection. DEB are composed of either a sulfonate-modified poly(vinyl alcohol) hydrogel (DC Bead®; Biocompatibles, Surrey, UK) or a sodium acrylate and vinyl alcohol copolymer (HepaSphere™; BioSphere Medical, Inc., Rockland, MA, USA). For the treatment of HCC, both particles can be loaded with doxorubicin. Significant reductions of peak plasma concentrations have been observed with DEB when compared with conventional chemoembolization, suggesting that a greater amount of the anticancer agent is being sequestered by the tumor versus being released in the systemic circulation [55]. With regard to their embolizing properties, DEB tend to produce a more distal occlusion than polyvinyl alcohol particles, and the rate of recanalization is considerably lower [11].

Clinical Evidence and Safety Profile

The first human reports on TACE with DEB in HCC [56, 57] supported the preclinical investigation and the results achieved in animal models, administering doses of up to 150 mg doxorubicin without relevant drug-related toxicity, consistent with reduced systemic exposure to the drug. Consistent objective response at a rate of 60–66.6% using the European Association for the Study of the Liver (EASL) criteria [57, 58] and of 70% according to mRECIST were reported [56].

Postembolization syndrome was observed in 41 and 18% of the treated patients after the first and the second treatment, respectively. There were two cases of liver abscesses in the series from Varela [57], and the treatment-related complication rate was 11% in the phase I–II study [56].

In a large, international randomized controlled trial comparing conventional TACE with DEB-TACE using DC Beads, primary endpoints (superiority of DEB-TACE in achieving objective tumor response at 6 months according to EASL criteria and in producing fewer treatment-related serious adverse events in the first 30 days) were not met. Tumor response rates were 52 and 44% and time to progression (TTP) was 7.1 and 6.4 months for DEB-TACE and conventional TACE, respectively. However, DEB-TACE produced a significantly higher response rate in a small subgroup of patients carrying the worst prognosis (e.g., those with Child-Pugh B, Eastern Cooperative Group Oncology (ECOG) 1, bilobar disease, and recurrent disease) and was associated with a significant reduction of doxorubicin-related side effects [59]. This potential advantage should be treated with caution as it comes from the analysis of a very small group of patients and as it is generally recognized that TACE should be indicated very stringently in this subgroup of patients who have a poor prognosis for which a survival advantage has not been shown after conventional TACE. Regarding the use of Hepa-Sphere, few data on HCC patients are available but a similar response rate of 51% at 6 months was reported in a multicenter study [60].

Malagari et al. [61] have reported on 173 patients prospectively enrolled and treated segmentally with DEB-TACE. All patients had underlying cirrhosis (Child-Pugh class A or B) and were in BCLC stages A (22%) and B (78%). The overall survival rate at 1, 3, and 5 years was 93.6, 62, and 22.5%. The majority of patients (74%) were observed to have varying degrees of self-limiting postembolization symptoms. Major complications occurred in 4.1% of the patients and included liver abscess, cholecystitis, pleural effusion, and three cases of irreversible liver failure [61].

The same authors conducted a prospective randomized comparison of DEB-TACE and bland embolization in 84 cirrhotic patients. The objective response rate according to EASL criteria was higher in the DEB-TACE group than in the bland embolization group at 9 months (55 vs. 31%). However, the survival rate at 12 months was similar in both groups (85.3% for the DEB-TACE group and 86% for the bland embolization group) [62].

The most recent data published to date comes from the Barcelona retrospective series [63]. A total of 104 well-compensated cirrhotic patients (95% with Child-Pugh A) were treated with DEB-TACE. After censoring for other treatments, the median overall survival was 40.6 months (95% confidence interval (CI): 12.8–84.4) in BCLC-A stage (40% of the patients) and 42.8 months (95% CI: 27.6–58.0) for BCLC-B stage (60% of the patients). However, the median follow-up was 24.5 months and therefore much shorter than the median survival, so this result warrants prolonged follow-up to be confirmed. In order to offer a larger standardization procedure, treatment frequency and schedule should be detailed. Major complications developed in 10% of the patients, and single treatment-related death was at 0.96%.

Combination with Systemic Agents

TACE potentially causes hypoxia in tumors as well as in surrounding liver tissues due to the anticancer effects of chemotherapy and embolization to feeding arteries. Ischemic injury after TACE can induce upregulation of circulating vascular endothelial growth factor (VEGF) [64], which is essential for HCC growth, invasion, and metastasis. Recent studies have reported a significant association between VEGF upregulation after TACE and poor prognosis [65, 66]. Therefore, adjuvant or concurrent use of an antiangiogenic agent may be helpful for HCC patients who are treated with TACE. TACE plus an antiangiogenic agent, such as sorafenib, could potentially provide complementary inhibition of angiogenic factors and tumor growth [67]. Combination strategies that have been proposed [67] include: i) a sequential schedule in which systemic therapy is started after all TACE sessions are completed, with an adjuvant intention to delay or block the growth of metastasis; ii) a continuous schedule in which systemic therapy is started before the first TACE session and maintained thereafter to provide better interference with the peak production of neoangiogenic factors after each session; and iii) an interrupted schedule in which systemic therapy is put on hold for a few days after each TACE session to reduce the chance of synergistic toxicity.

Several clinical trials are currently evaluating the effect of conventional TACE or DEB-TACE with systemic agents on the outcome of patients with unresectable HCC, using all three schedules [68]. The results of three of these randomized controlled trials are already available. Kudo et al. [69] failed to show an improvement in TTP among patients with unresectable HCC in Child-Pugh A stage with >25% tumor necrosis or shrinkage at 1–3 months following one or two TACE sessions that received sorafenib when compared to those that received placebo (5.4 vs. 3.7 months; $p = 0.25$). Overall survival was not significantly different between groups. The two other phase II trials were aimed to assess the safety of the combination of sorafenib with conventional TACE [70] or with DEB-TACE [71]. Both trials showed a safe profile, with most adverse events being related to sorafenib and manageable with dose modifications. Preliminary data from the SPACE study (NCT 00494299) were presented at the American Society of Clinical Oncology [72]. This phase II study explored the combination of a continuous regimen of sorafenib with DEB-TACE versus DEB-TACE alone, with TTP as primary endpoint. The hazard ratio for TTP was 0.797 (95% CI: 0.588–1.080; $p = 0.072$). Although this preliminary efficacy data are encouraging, definitive results of ongoing, large phase III trials (ECOG study – NCT 01004978) are needed to confirm these results.

Radioembolization

Technical Considerations

The term radioembolization (90Y-RE) was proposed by a group of experts to define those procedures in which intra-arterially injected radioactive microspheres are used for internal radiation treatment (mainly in the liver) [73]. The term selective internal radiation therapy (SIRT) has been widely used to name these procedures but it may be confusing since non-transarterial techniques such as high-dose-rate interstitial brachytherapy also provide selective internal radiation.

There are different radioactive isotopes used for the treatment of liver tumors; however, 90Y is the one most commonly utilized due to its specific properties as a pure beta emitter, with a half-life of 64.2 h and a short tissue penetration (mean:

2.5 mm). Consequently, isolation for radiation protection is not needed following treatment. There are two types of commercially available radioactive microspheres: 90Y glass microspheres (TheraSphere®; MDS Nordion, Ottawa, ON, Canada) and 90Y resin microspheres (SIR-Spheres®; Sirtex Medical Limited, Sydney, Australia). Beyond the differences in the materials used for each type of microspheres, these devices differ in the amount of radioactive isotope loaded in each microsphere (larger for glass microspheres), which in turn determines the number of microspheres typically injected in a single treatment (smaller for glass microspheres).

In TACE, particles larger than 100 microns are used to occlude tumor-feeding vessels in order to produce ischemia and to increase the drug exposure of tumor cells. 90Y-RE does not produce an occlusion of large- or medium-sized arteries, and the smaller particles used in radioembolization (20–60 mm) reach the tumor microvasculature, and therefore, high doses of radiation are delivered preferentially to tumor tissues. The efficacy and toxicity of the treatment are thus a consequence of radiation and to some extent of microembolization, but are not due to ischemia.

A simulation of the actual treatment is performed 1–2 weeks prior to radioembolization. It consists of a thorough angiographic evaluation to detect extrahepatic vessels irrigating liver tumors as well as to detect, and to eventually occlude, aberrant vessels arising from hepatic arteries that may feed the gastrointestinal tract (mainly gastroduodenal artery and right gastric artery). During this arteriography, technetium-99m-labeled macroaggregated albumin (99mTc-MAA) is injected as a tracer. 99mTc-MAA allows for planar and/or SPECT gamma-camera imaging, which can be used to measure hepatopulmonary shunting and to anticipate an average dose of radiation that could be delivered to tumor areas. Patients can only be considered for 90Y-RE provided that the degree of arteriovenous shunting to the lung is limited, that there is no possibility of microspheres potentially reaching the gastrointestinal tract, and that the liver has had no prior exposure to external irradiation [73]. Liver function must be adequate, without ascites or hepatic encephalopathy, and with a total bilirubin <2 mg/dl [74].

Clinical Evidence

All the evidence comes from retrospective series or non-controlled prospective studies [41, 75–82] without any randomized controlled trials comparing 90Y-RE with other available therapies. However, in the last 3 years four large series have provided valuable information for the different stages of HCC and may allow putting the outcomes in the perspective of other treatments, mainly in terms of survival [82–86]. Besides, some of these series provide data on toxicity and on surrogate endpoints that are likely to predict clinical benefit, such as objective tumor response rates and TTP. Despite this growing body of evidence and due to the lack of randomized controlled trials, 90Y-RE is not recommended in the proposed algorithms of treatment in the EASL and AASLD (American Association for the Study of Liver Diseases) guidelines [2, 22]. However, its use is considered in other guidelines such as those by the European Society for Medical Oncology (ESMO) [87] and the National Comprehensive Cancer Network (NCCN) [88].

First reports in the literature mainly included the application of 90Y-RE for the treatment of unresectable advanced HCC. In the last years, as its use has been extended, some series have reported the outcomes of 90Y-RE in early tumors.

90Y-RE can induce complete necrosis in targeted lesions, as has been suggested by the analyses of 35 explanted livers from patients treated with 90Y-RE, as a bridge or after successful downstaging to liver transplantation. Nearly 90% of the tumors up to 3 cm in size and two-thirds of those between 3 and 5 cm had a complete pathologic necrosis [89].

In terms of survival, recent series describing outcomes according to tumor stage have reported a consistent median overall survival of around 26 months [35, 83, 84] in patients at early stages (inoperable BCLC-A) after 90Y-RE. This survival is in between the wide range of median survival from 16.8 to 45.4 months reported with TACE/transarterial embolization (TAE) in large series of BCLC-A patients, as previously described [31–36, 63]. Median TTP in this early stage has been described as long as 25.1 months (95% CI: 8–27 months), i.e., longer than the one observed with TACE in a retrospective, well-balanced comparative study between both techniques (TACE and 90Y-RE) [35], and this may provide a rationale for its use as a bridge to liver transplantation in an attempt to avoid dropping from the waiting list [90].

The potential to induce intense tumor responses has allowed 90Y-RE to be used as a downstaging therapy, to reduce the tumor burden within acceptable limits for liver transplantation, to render non-operable patients operable, or to simplify surgery. Besides tumor response, atrophy of the radiated lobe after 90Y-RE and contralateral lobe hypertrophy as a result of the injection of a high-activity 90Y in a lobar hepatic artery, known as 'radiation lobectomy', may contribute to resectability [91]. In the largest series published with 90Y glass microspheres for downstaging HCC to radical therapies, 23 of 35 patients (66%) achieved resection, radiofrequency ablation (RFA), T2 status, or transplant, although 8 of these patients (23%) chose close observation rather than RFA or transplantation, and the 1- and 3-year survival rates achieved were 84 and 27%, respectively [69]. Compared with TACE, downstaging from T3 to T2 was achieved more frequently with 90Y-RE (58 vs. 31%; $p = 0.023$), and overall survival was in favor of 90Y-RE (censored: 35.7 vs. 18.7 months for TACE, $p = 0.18$; uncensored: 41.6 vs. 19.2 months, $p = 0.008$, respectively) [80]. Our group has also analyzed the potential of downstaging HCC with 90Y resin microspheres in patients in T3 stage treated for palliative intent. Overall, 29% of 21 UNOS

Table 2. Median survival according to the presence or absence of portal vein thrombosis (PVT) and extrahepatic disease (EHD) with ^{90}Y-RE and conventional TACE

	Author, year [reference]	PVT			
		yes		no	
		number of patients	median survival, months (95% CI)	number of patients	median survival, months (95% CI)
^{90}Y-RE	Kulik et al., 2008 [80]	12 main PVT	4.4 (2.9–7.5)	71	15.5 (10.7–20.9)
		25 branch PVT	10.1 (7.2–16)		
	Iñarrairaegui et al., 2010 [81]	25 (72% branch PVT)	10 (6.6–13.3)		
	Hilgard et al., 2010 [84]	33 (50% branch PVT)	10 (6–∞)	75	16.4 (12.1–∞)
	Woodall et al., 2009 [101]	15 (73% main PVT)	3.2	20	13.9
	Sangro et al., 2011 [84]	76 (58% branch PVT)	10.0 (6.5–11.8)	249	15.3 (12.4–18.4)
	Mazzaferro et al., 2013 [86]	29 branch or segmental PVT	14 (11–18)	17	18 (12.0–38.0)
		6 main PVT	8 (5–8)		
TACE	Luo et al., 2011 [42]	44 main PVT	5.3		
		40 branch PVT	10.2		
		EHD			
		yes		no	
		number of patients	median survival, months (95% CI)	number of patients	median survival, months (95% CI)
^{90}Y-RE	Sangro et al., 2011 [85]	30	7.4 (4.8–13–1)	295	14.1 (11.7–16.8)
	Salem et al., 2011 [35]	45	5.4 (2.7–7.5)	107 (BCLC-C)	7.3 (6.5–10.1)

(United Network for Organ Sharing) T3 stage patients were downstaged and underwent surgical resection or liver transplantation, with a 3-year survival rate of 75% [92], which is comparable with the survival of patients with early-stage disease who are treated radically at the time of diagnosis.

BCLC stage B patients treated with 90Y-RE have reached a median survival ranging between 16.4 and 18 months [83, 85, 86], comparable with the median survival achieved by TACE in this stage (15.6–18.2 months) [31–34, 36]. These findings are confirmed by retrospective analyses of different stages of HCC treated with TACE or 90Y-RE at the same institution in which nearly equivalent survivals between these treatments were found [35, 93–95]. Salem et al. [35] have reported the compared outcomes of patients that did not show PVT or extrahepatic disease. This series mainly included patients with intermediate (53%) or early (35%) tumors treated in the same period (2001–2010) in which treatment allocation was decided by a multidisciplinary team. When patients in the intermediate stage were evaluated separately, an identical survival rate in the intermediate stage was observed after each treatment (15.5 vs. 17.2 months).

Besides, not all patients with intermediate-stage HCC are considered good candidates for TACE as those patients with a bulky disease or one affecting both lobes are widely regarded as poor candidates [54]. In this subgroup of intermediate patients, 90Y-RE can improve survival compared with either experimental therapies or best supportive care (16 vs. 8 months; $p < 0.05$), as shown by a case-control study [96], and is similar to the median survival of 14.5 months achieved in the sorafenib arm of BCLC stage B patients of the SHARP (Sorafenib HCC Assessment Randomized Protocol) trial [97]. For patients who fail to respond to TACE, the only remaining treatment options are either sorafenib or 90Y-RE. In a subset analysis of SHARP studies, survival in patients failing TACE was 11.9 and 9.9 months for the sorafenib and the placebo treatment arms, respectively [97]. By comparison, investigators from the European Network on Radioembolization with 90Y resin microspheres (ENRY) found that survival was 11.4 months for a subset of usual candidates for 90Y-RE (matching the SHARP criteria) and 15.4 months in BCLC-B patients failing TACE/TAE [85].

Sorafenib is the mainstay for treating advanced HCC, defined by the presence of vascular invasion, extrahepatic disease, or deteriorated performance status in a patient with at least partially preserved liver function. As 90Y-RE has no macroembolic effect [98, 99], it can be successfully applied to patients with PVT and can offer a similar median survival in the range of 6 to 13 months [83–86], being very akin to the 6.5–10.7 months reported in the phase III clinical trials of sorafenib in the same group of patients [100, 101]. However, one must take into account that the extent of PVT also matters. When thrombosis affects the main trunk, survival is more disappointing and ranges between 3.2 and 8 months [80, 86, 102], while survival extends to 10–14 months in patients with branch thrombosis only (table 2) [80, 81, 86].

Metastases are not the direct cause of death in the majority of HCC patients; thus, a locoregional treatment may be considered when a small metastatic burden involves non-vital organs such as bone, adrenal glands, or lymph nodes. Nevertheless, extrahepatic disease is an indicator of disease aggressiveness [102], and median survival in metastatic patients treated with 90Y-RE is poor, ranging between 5.4 and 7.4 months [83, 85].

Safety Profile

The toxicity profile of 90Y-RE is favorable and treatment is generally well tolerated. A postembolization syndrome like the one that appears after TACE is not seen; however, in large series several rather mild procedure-related symptoms, including fatigue (54–61%), abdominal pain (23–56%), nausea and vomiting (20–32%), and low-grade fever (3–12%), may ensue that usually last only a few hours [83–86]. Potentially more serious adverse events resulting from irradiation of non-tumoral tissues include pneumonitis [103], cholecystitis [104], gastrointestinal ulceration [105], and liver damage, but these events are uncommon.

Liver toxicity after 90Y-RE is the most challenging adverse event in HCC patients as the majority of these tumors arise in cirrhotic livers, with some degree of reduced functional reserve. However, it is sometimes difficult to differentiate between the liver damage due to the treatment with 90Y-RE and the deterioration of liver function as a consequence of disease progression of the liver disease. A comprehensive analysis of the data in the literature is hampered by the wide variations between the patient series in the timing of liver function testing after 90Y-RE, in the populations treated, and in the toxicity criteria used. Hyperbilirubinemia has been reported in 3–40% [76, 77, 80, 84, 101, 104], while hypertransaminasemia or elevation of cholestasis enzymes has been described between 0 and 80% [76, 77, 84, 85, 104, 106]. Signs of liver dysfunction, such as ascites (0–18%) or encephalopathy (0–4%), also vary between series [76, 77, 80, 84, 101, 104]. The only group that has published specific liver toxicity induced by 90Y-RE has described in non-cirrhotic livers a clinical syndrome characterized by jaundice, mild ascites, and a moderate increase in GGT and alkaline phosphatase, histopathologically similar to a sinusoidal obstruction syndrome, which is called radioembolization-induced liver disease (REILD) [107]. Its incidence in cirrhotic patients was 9.3% in the largest series reported so far [108].

Safety is a special issue in patients with compromised liver flow, similar to those with PVT. In the first and largest series published by the Chicago group, patients with cirrhosis and PVT involving the main trunk had a higher incidence of adverse events (a non-statistically significant increment in bilirubin levels and a significant increase in ascites) [80]. The ENRY series analyzed main clinical adverse events and liver toxicity in the different BCLC stages and observed similar liver toxicity across BCLC stages A through C [85]. Compared to those with intermediate or early stage disease, only fatigue was most commonly reported in the advanced stage (61.2%), which is not surprising since fatigue is usually associated with altered performance status. Finally, no significant differences in toxicity were registered when patients with and without PVT were compared in the Milan phase II trial [86].

Despite an intense local effect of 90Y-RE on target lesions, progression is usually the result of the growth of new liver lesions, particularly in those patients with more advanced disease. New lesions arise as frequently in the targeted areas as in the non-targeted areas of the liver, reflecting the irrelevant therapeutic effect of Y90-RE on HCC micrometastases, probably due to their poor arterial blood supply. And importantly, the early appearance of new lesions has prognostic relevance since these patients have a much worse prognosis.

The combination of systemic therapy with sorafenib and 90Y-RE is being investigated in two trials, i.e. SORAMIC (NCT 01126645) and STOP-HCC (NCT 01556490), with survival as primary endpoint in non-resectable HCC patients. Finally, two head-to-head comparisons of sorafenib versus 90Y-RE with survival as the primary endpoint are now ongoing (SIRveNIB – NCT 01135056; SARAH – NCT 01482442).

Conclusion

TACE is in fact a very heterogeneous group of procedures that is actually performed in very different ways regarding materials, extent and selectivity of vessel occlusion, and timing of repeated sessions. Good results are generally observed when a reduced number of not very large tumors are embolized in a selective fashion (ideally through a distinct feeding vessel). In the past few years, DEB-TACE has become a reproducible and well-tolerated procedure associated with low complication as well as promising tumor response rates and is a valuable alternative to conventional TACE in some centers. However, all clinical trials conducted so far have failed to show an advantage of DEB-TACE over conventional TACE regarding response rate or overall survival. Secondary endpoints including reduction of drug-related adverse events or increased intratumoral necrosis (which makes the difference between RECIST and EASL criteria) have been successfully proven and are consistent with the well-known characteristics of the beads as shown in preclinical work.

Y90-RE is a form of brachytherapy for liver tumors in which the source of radiation has to access the network of tumoral neovessels after having been injected into the hepatic arteries. Evidence supporting the usefulness of 90Y-RE in the treatment of HCC patients is derived from non-controlled series. Most information comes from patients with advanced HCC who are not suitable for other locoregional therapies or who have failed in TACE. In recent years, however, encouraging experience has been reported in the treatment of HCC patients at earlier stages, including those in which downstaging is likely to be beneficial. There is a group of patients for which the benefit of being treated with 90Y-RE is unlikely or needs to be further substantiated. This group includes patients with diffuse bulky disease involving more than 50% of liver volume as well as patients with a tumoral thrombosis of the main portal trunk and a poor liver functional reserve.

Due to the lack of randomized controlled trials comparing both techniques, it is a difficult question to answer how Y90-RE does compare to TACE in the same patient population. For those patients with small- to medium-sized tumors that can be treated selectively, TACE is certainly the standard of care and can be provided in most centers. Y90-RE could then be an alternative to repeated TACE for patients who fail to respond to initial TACE and a first option for those who are poor candidates for TACE, mainly because of bulky disease and PVT, but who still have a good liver function.

In the next years, much attention is likely to be paid to the combination of targeted agents with antiangiogenic activity and locoregional therapies. The results of the ongoing clinical trials will establish the best way of combining sorafenib and other targeted therapies with locoregional procedures, including TACE and Y90-RE.

Disclosure Statement

Mercedes Iñarraíraegui and Delia D'Avola do not have any financial disclosures. Bruno Sangro receives lecture fees from Sirtex Medical Europe GmBH and Bayer Health Care.

References

1 Bosch FX, Ribes J, Diaz M, et al: Primary liver cancer: worldwide incidence and trends. Gastroenterology 2004;127:S5–S16.
2 European Association For The Study Of The Liver; European Organisation For Research And Treatment Of Cancer: EASL-EORTC clinical practice guidelines: management of hepatocellular carcinoma. J Hepatol 2012;56:908–943.
3 Bolondi L, Sofia S, Siringo S, et al: Surveillance programme of cirrhotic patients for early diagnosis and treatment of hepatocellular carcinoma: a cost-effectiveness analysis. Gut 2001;48:251–259.
4 Sangiovanni A, Del Ninno E, Fasani P, et al: Increased survival of cirrhotic patients with a hepatocellular carcinoma detected during surveillance. Gastroenterology 2004;126:1005–1014.
5 Kim WR, Gores GJ, Benson JT, et al: Mortality and hospital utilization for hepatocellular carcinoma in the United States. Gastroenterology 2005;129:486–493.
6 Marelli L, Stigliano R, Triantos C, et al: Transarterial therapy for hepatocellular carcinoma: which technique is more effective? A systematic review of cohort and randomized studies. Cardiovasc Intervent Radiol 2007;30:6–25.
7 Nakamura H, Hashimoto T, Oi H, et al: Transcatheter oily chemoembolization of hepatocellular carcinoma. Radiology 1989;170:783–786.
8 Raoul JL, Heresbach D, Bretagne JF, et al: Chemoembolization of hepatocellular carcinomas. A study of the biodistribution and pharmacokinetics of doxorubicin. Cancer 1992;70:585–590.
9 Kan Z, McCuskey PA, Wright KC, et al: Role of Kupffer cells in iodized oil embolization. Invest Radiol 1994;29:990–993.
10 Coldwell DM, Stokes KR, Yakes WF: Embolotherapy: agents, clinical applications, and techniques. Radiographics 1994;14:623–643.
11 Bilbao JI, de Luis E, Garcia de Jalon JA, et al: Comparative study of four different spherical embolic particles in an animal model: a morphologic and histologic evaluation. J Vasc Interv Radiol 2008;12:1625–1638.
12 Kruskal JB, Hlatky L, Hahnfeldt P, et al: In vivo and in vitro analysis of the effectiveness of doxorubicin combined with temporary arterial occlusion in liver tumors. J Vasc Interv Radiol 1993;4:741–747.
13 Chang JM, Tzeng WS, Pan HB, et al: Transcatheter arterial embolization with or without cisplatin treatment of hepatocellular carcinoma. A randomized controlled study. Cancer 1994;74:2449–2453.
14 Kawai S, Okamura J, Ogawa M, et al: Prospective and randomized clinical trial for the treatment of hepatocellular carcinoma – a comparison of lipiodol-transcatheter arterial embolization with and without adriamycin (first cooperative study). The cooperative study group for liver cancer treatment of Japan. Cancer Chemother Pharmacol 1992;31(suppl):S1–6.
15 Cammà C, Schepis F, Orlando A, et al: Transarterial chemoembolization for unresectable hepatocellular carcinoma: meta-analysis of randomized controlled trials. Radiology 2002;224:47–54.
16 Llovet JM, Real MI, Montaña X, et al: Arterial embolisation or chemoembolisation versus symptomatic treatment in patients with unresectable hepatocellular carcinoma: a randomized controlled trial. Lancet 2002;359:1734–1739.
17 Lo CM, Ngan H, Tso WK, et al: Randomized controlled trial of transarterial lipiodol chemoembolization for unresectable hepatocellular carcinoma. Hepatology 2002;35:1164–1171.
18 A comparison of lipiodol chemoembolization and conservative treatment for unresectable hepatocellular carcinoma. Groupe d'etude et de traitement du carcinoma hepatocellulaire. N Engl J Med 1995;332:1256–1261.
19 Pelletier G, Ducreux M, Gay F, et al: Treatment of unresectable hepatocellular carcinoma with lipiodol chemoembolization: a multicenter randomized trial. Groupe CHC. J Hepatol 1998;29:129–134.
20 Doffoel M, Bonnetain F, Bouche O, et al: Multicentre randomised phase III trial comparing tamoxifen alone or with transarterial lipiodol chemoembolization for unresectable hepatocellular carcinoma in cirrhotic patients (federation francophone de cancerologie digestive 9402). Eur J Cancer 2008;44:528–538.
21 Llovet J, Bruix J: Systematic review of randomized trials for unresectable hepatocellular carcinoma: chemoembolization improves survival. Hepatology 2003;37:429–442.
22 Bruix J, Sherman M: Management of hepatocellular carcinoma: an update. Hepatology 2011;53:1020–1022.
23 Takayasu K, Arii S, Ikai I, et al: Prospective cohort study of transarterial chemoembolization for unresectable hepatocellular carcinoma in 8510 patients. Gastroenterology 2006;131:461–469.
24 Poon RT, Ngan H, Lo CM, et al: Transarterial chemoembolization for inoperable hepatocellular carcinoma and postresection intrahepatic recurrence. J Surg Oncol 2000;73:109–114.
25 O'Suilleabhain CB, Poon RT, Yong JL, et al: Factors predictive of 5-year survival after transarterial chemoembolization for inoperable hepatocellular carcinoma. Br J Surg 2003;90:325–331.
26 Katyal S, Oliver JH, Peterson MS, et al: Prognostic significance of arterial phase CT for prediction of response to transcatheter arterial chemoembolization in unresectable hepatocellular carcinoma: a retrospective analysis. AJR Am J Roentgenol 2000;175:1665–1672.
27 Bronowicki JP, Vetter D, Dumas F, et al: Transcatheter oily chemoembolization for hepatocellular carcinoma. A 4-year study of 127 French patients. Cancer 1994;74:16–24.
28 Herber SC, Otto G, Schneider J, et al: Transarterial chemoembolization in patients not eligible for liver transplantation: single-center results. AJR Am J Roentgenol 2008;190:1035–1042.
29 Barone M, Ettorre GC, Ladisa R, et al: Transcatheter arterial chemoembolization (TACE) in treatment of hepatocellular carcinoma. Hepatogastroenterology 2003;50:183–187.
30 Llado L, Virgili J, Figueras J, et al: A prognostic index of the survival of patients with unresectable hepatocellular carcinoma after transcatheter arterial chemoembolization. Cancer 2000;88:50–57.
31 Chen CH, Hu FC, Huang GT, et al: Applicability of staging systems for patients with hepatocellular carcinoma is dependent on treatment method analysis of 2010 Taiwanese patients. Eur J Cancer 2009;45:1630–1639.
32 Hsu KF, Chu CH, Chan DC, et al: Superselective transarterial chemoembolization vs hepatic resection for resectable early-stage hepatocellular carcinoma in patients with Child-Pugh class a liver function. Eur J Radiol 2011;81:466–471.
33 Ho MC, Huang GT, Tsang YM, et al: Liver resection improves survival of patients with multiple hepatocellular carcinomas. Ann Surg Oncol 2009;16:848–855.

34 Lewandowski RJ, Mulcahy MF, Kulik LM, et al: Chemoembolization for hepatocellular carcinoma: comprehensive imaging and survival analysis in a 172-patient cohort. Radiology 2010;255:955–965.
35 Salem R, Lewandowski RJ, Kulik L, et al: Radioembolization results in longer time-to-progression and reduced toxicity compared with chemoembolization in patients with hepatocellular carcinoma. Gastroenterology 2011;140:497–507.
36 Wang JH, Changchien CS, Hu TH, et al: The efficacy of treatment schedules according to Barcelona Clinic Liver Cancer staging for hepatocellular carcinoma – survival analysis of 3892 patients. Eur J Cancer 2008;44:1000–1006.
37 Farinati F, De Maria N, Marafin C, et al: Unresectable hepatocellular carcinoma in cirrhosis: survival, prognostic factors, and unexpected side effects after transcatheter arterial chemoembolization. Dig Dis Sci 1996;41:2332–2339.
38 Chen MS, Li JQ, Zhang YQ, et al: High-dose iodized oil transcatheter arterial chemoembolization for patients with large hepatocellular carcinoma. World J Gastroenterol 2002;8:74–78.
39 Huo T, Huang YH, Wu JC, et al: Comparison of transarterial chemoembolization and percutaneous acetic acid injection as the primary loco-regional therapy for unresectable hepatocellular carcinoma: a prospective survey. Aliment Pharmacol Ther 2004;19:1301–1308.
40 Nouso K, Ito Y, Kuwaki K, et al: Prognostic factors and treatment effects for hepatocellular carcinoma in child C cirrhosis. Br J Cancer 2008;98:1161–1165.
41 Lewandowski RJ, Kulik LM, Riaz A, et al: A comparative analysis of transarterial downstaging for hepatocellular carcinoma: chemoembolization versus radioembolization. Am J Transplant 2009;9: 1920–1928.
42 Luo J, Guo RP, Lai EC, et al: Transarterial chemoembolization for unresectable hepatocellular carcinoma with portal vein tumor thrombosis: a prospective comparative study. Ann Surg Oncol 2011; 18:413–420.
43 Kim KM, Kim JH, Park IS, et al: Reappraisal of repeated transarterial chemoembolization in the treatment of hepatocellular carcinoma with portal vein invasion. J Gastroenterol Hepatol 2009;24:806–814.
44 Wigmore SJ, Redhead DN, Thomson BN, et al: Postchemoembolisation syndrome – tumour necrosis or hepatocyte injury? Br J Cancer 2003;89: 1423–1427.
45 Chan A, Yuen MF, Hui CK, et al: A prospective study regarding the complications of transcatheter intraarterial lipiodol chemoembolization in patients with hepatocellular carcinoma. Cancer 2002; 94:1747–1752.
46 Castells A, Bruix J, Ayuso C, et al: Transarterial embolization for hepatocellular carcinoma. Antibiotic prophylaxis and clinical meaning of postembolization fever. J Hepatol 1995;22:410–415.
47 Chung JW, Park JH, Han JK, et al: Hepatic tumors: predisposing factors for complications of transcatheter oily chemoembolization. Radiology 1996;198:33–40.
48 Pietrosi G, Miraglia R, Luca A, et al: Arterial chemoembolization/embolization and early complications after hepatocellular carcinoma treatment: a safe standardized protocol in selected patients with child class A and B cirrhosis. J Vasc Interv Radiol 2009;20:896–902.
49 Kim HK, Chung YH, Song BC, et al: Ischemic bile duct injury as a serious complication after transarterial chemoembolization in patients with hepatocellular carcinoma. J Clin Gastroenterol 2001;32: 423–427.
50 Yu JS, Kim KW, Jeong MG, et al: Predisposing factors of bile duct injury after transcatheter arterial chemoembolization (TACE) for hepatic malignancy. Cardiovasc Intervent Radiol 2002;25:270–274.
51 Chen JH, Ho YJ, Shen WC: Asymptomatic arteriobiliary fistula after transarterial chemoembolization of metastatic liver tumors. Hepatogastroenterology 2001;48:842–843.
52 Leung TK, Lee CM, Chen HC: Anatomic and technical skill factor of gastroduodenal complication in post-transarterial embolization for hepatocellular carcinoma: a retrospective study of 280 cases. World J Gastroenterol 2005;11:1554–1557.
53 Shi M, Chen JA, Lin XJ, et al: Transarterial chemoembolization as initial treatment for unresectable hepatocellular carcinoma in southern China. World J Gastroenterol 2010;16:264–269.
54 Raoul JL, Sangro B, Forner A, et al: Evolving strategies for the management of intermediate-stage hepatocellular carcinoma: available evidence and expert opinion on the use of transarterial chemoembolization. Cancer Treat Rev 2011;37: 212–220.
55 Hong K, Khwaja A, Liapi E, et al: New intra-arterial drug delivery system for the treatment of liver cancer: preclinical assessment in a rabbit model. Clin Cancer Res 2006;12:2563–2567.
56 Poon RT, Tso WK, Pang RW, et al: A phase I/II trial of chemoembolization for hepatocellular carcinoma using a novel intra-arterial drug-eluting bead. Clin Gastroenterol Hepatol 2007;5:1100–1108.
57 Varela M, Real MI, Burrel M, et al: Chemoembolization of hepatocellular carcinoma with drug eluting beads: efficacy and doxorubicin pharmacokinetics. J Hepatol 2007;46:474–481.
58 Reyes DK, Vossen JA, Kamel IR, et al: Single-center phase II trial of transarterial chemoembolization with drug-eluting beads for patients with unresectable hepatocellular carcinoma: initial experience in the United States. Cancer J 2009;15: 526–532.
59 Lammer J, Malagari K, Vogl T, et al: Prospective randomized study of doxorubicin-eluting-bead embolization in the treatment of hepatocellular carcinoma: results of the PRECISION V study. Cardiovasc Intervent Radiol 2010;33:41–52.
60 Grosso M, Vignali C, Quaretti P, et al: Transarterial chemoembolization for hepatocellular carcinoma with drug-eluting microspheres: preliminary results from an Italian multicentre study. Cardiovasc Intervent Radiol 2008;31:1141–1149.
61 Malagari K, Pomoni M, Moschouris H, et al: Chemoembolization with doxorubicin eluting beads for unresectable hepatocellular carcinoma: five-year survival analysis. Cardiovasc Intervent Radiol 2012;35:1119–1128.
62 Malagari K, Pomoni M, Kelekis A, et al: Prospective randomized comparison of chemoembolization with doxorubicin-eluting beads and bland embolization with BeadBlock for hepatocellular carcinoma. Cardiovasc Intervent Radiol 2010;33:541–551.
63 Burrel M, Reig M, Forner A, et al: Survival of patients with hepatocelllular carcinoma treated by transarterial chemoembolisation (TACE) using Drug Eluting Beads. Implications for clinical practice and trial design. J Hepatol 2012;56:1330–1335.
64 Li X, Feng GS, Zheng CS, Zhuo CK, Liu X: Expression of plasma vascular endothelial growth factor in patients with hepatocellular carcinoma and effect of transcatheter arterial chemoembolization therapy on plasma vascular endothelial growth factor level. World J Gastroenterol 2004;10:2878–2882.
65 Shim JH, Park JW, Kim JH, et al: Association between increment of serum VEGF level and prognosis after transcatheter arterial chemoembolization in hepatocellular carcinoma patients. Cancer Sci 2008;99:2037–2044.
66 Sergio A, Cristofori C, Cardin R, et al: Transcatheter arterial chemoembolization (TACE) in hepatocellular carcinoma (HCC): the role of angiogenesis and invasiveness. Am J Gastroenterol 2008; 103:914–921.
67 Strebel BM, Dufour JF: Combined approach to hepatocellular carcinoma: a new treatment concept for nonresectable disease. Expert Rev Anticancer Ther 2008;8:1743–1749.
68 *www.clinicaltrials.gov/ct2/results?term = hepatocellular +carcinoma+TACE+sorafenib.*
69 Kudo M, Imanaka K, Chida N, et al: Phase III study of sorafenib after transarterial chemoembolisation in Japanese and Korean patients with unresectable hepatocellular carcinoma. Eur J Cancer 2011;47:2117–2127.
70 Park JW, Koh YH, Kim HB, et al: Phase II study of concurrent transarterial chemoembolization and sorafenib in patients with unresectable hepatocellular carcinoma. J Hepatol 2012;56:1336–1342.
71 Pawlik TM, Reyes DK, Cosgrove D, et al: Phase II trial of sorafenib combined with concurrent transarterial chemoembolization with drug-eluting beads for hepatocellular carcinoma. J Clin Oncol 2011;29: 3960–3967.
72 Lencioni R, Llovet JM, Han G, et al: Sorafenib or placebo in combination with transarterial chemoembolization (TACE) with doxorubicin-eluting beads (DEBDOX) for intermediate-stage hepatocellular carcinoma: phase II, randomized, double-blind SPACE trial. J Clin Oncol 2012;30(suppl 4): LBA 154.
73 Kennedy A, Nag S, Salem R, et al: Recommendations for radioembolization of hepatic malignancies using yttrium-90 micorsphere brachiterapy: a consensus panel report from the radioembolization brachyterapy oncology conssortium. Int J Radiat Oncol Biol Phys 2007;68:13–23.
74 Coldwell D, Sangro B, Wasan H, et al: General selection criteria of patients for radioembolization of liver tumors: an international working group report. Am J Clin Oncol 2011;34:337–341.
75 Lau W, Leung W, Ho S, et al: Treatment of hepatocellular carcinoma with intra-hepatic arterial yttrium-90 microspheres: a phase I and II study. Br J Cancer 1994;70:994–999.
76 Geschwind JF, Salem R, Carr BI, et al: Yttrium-90 microspheres for the treatment of hepatocellular carcinoma. Gastroenterology 2004;127:S194–205.
77 Salem R, Lewandowski RJ, Atassi B, et al: Treatment of unresectable hepatocellular carcinoma with use of 90Y microspheres (TheraSphere): safety, tumor response, and survival. J Vasc Interv Radiol 2005;16:1627–1639.
78 Sangro B, Bilbao JI, Boan J, et al: Radioembolization using 90Y-resin microspheres for patients with advanced hepatocellular carcinoma. Int J Radiat Oncol Biol Phys 2006;66:792–800.
79 Kulik LM, Atassi B, van Holsbeeck L, et al: Yttrium-90 microspheres (TheraSphere) treatment of unresectable hepatocellular carcinoma: downstaging to resection, RFA and bridge to transplantation. J Surg Oncol 2006;94:572–586.
80 Kulik LM, Carr BI, Mulcahy MF, et al: Safety and efficacy of 90Y radiotherapy for hepatocellular carcinoma with and without portal vein thrombosis. Hepatology 2008;47:71–81.

81 Iñarrairaegui M, Thurston KG, Bilbao JI, et al: Radioembolization with use of yttrium-90 resin microspheres in patients with hepatocellular carcinoma and portal vein thrombosis. J Vasc Interv Radiol 2010;21:1205–1212.
82 Iñarrairaegui M, Martinez-Cuesta A, Rodríguez M, et al: Analysis of prognostic factors after yttrium-90 radioembolization of advanced hepatocellular carcinoma. Int J Radiat Oncol Biol Phys 2010;77: 1441–1448.
83 Salem R, Lewandowski RJ, Mulcahy MF, et al: Radioembolization for hepatocellular carcinoma using Yttrium-90 microspheres: a comprehensive report of long-term outcomes. Gastroenterology 2010;138:52–64.
84 Hilgard P, Hamami M, Fouly AE, et al: Radioembolization with yttrium-90 glass microspheres in hepatocellular carcinoma: European experience on safety and long-term survival. Hepatology 2010;52: 1741–1749.
85 Sangro B, Carpanese L, Cianni R; on behalf of the European Network on Radioembolization with Yttrium-90 Resin Microspheres (ENRY): Survival after Yttrium-90 resin microsphere radioembolization of hepatocellular carcinoma across Barcelona clinic liver cancer stages: a European evaluation. Hepatology 2011;54:868–878.
86 Mazzaferro V, Sposito C, Bhoori S, et al: Yttrium90 radioembolization for intermediate-advanced hepatocarcinoma: a phase II study. Hepatology 2012;DOI: 10.1002/hep.26014.
87 Jelic S, Sotiropoulos GC; ESMO Guidelines Working Group: Hepatocellular carcinoma: ESMO Clinical Practice Guidelines for diagnosis, treatment and follow-up. Ann Oncol 2010;21(suppl 5):v59–64.
88 Benson AB, Abrams TA, Ben-Josef E: NCCN clinical practice guidelines in oncology: hepatobiliary cancers. J Natl Compr Canc Netw 2009;7:350–391.
89 Riaz A, Kulik L, Lewandowski RJ, et al: Radiologic-pathologic correlation of hepatocellular carcinoma treated with internal radiation using yttrium-90 microspheres. Hepatology 2009;49:1185–1193.
90 Heckman JT, Devera MB, Marsh JW, et al: Bridging locoregional therapy for hepatocellular carcinoma prior to liver transplantation. Ann Surg Oncol 2008;15:3169–3177.
91 Gaba RC, Lewandowski RJ, Kulik LM, et al: Radiation lobectomy: preliminary findings of hepatic volumetric response to lobar yttrium-90 radioembolization. Ann Surg Oncol 2009;16:1587–1596.
92 Iñarrairaegui M, Pardo F, Bilbao JI, et al: Response to radioembolization with yttrium-90 resin microspheres may allow surgical treatment with curative intent and prolonged survival in previously unresectable hepatocellular carcinoma. Eur J Surg Oncol 2012;38:594–601.
93 Carr BI, Kondragunta V, Buch SC, et al: Therapeutic equivalence in survival for hepatic arterial chemoembolization and yttrium-90 microsphere treatments in unresectable hepatocellular carcinoma: a two cohort study. Cancer 2010;116: 1305–1314.
94 Kooby DA, Egnatashvili V, Srinivasan S, et al: Comparison of yttrium-90 radioembolization and transcatheter arterial chemoembolization for the treatment of unresectable hepatocellular carcinoma. J Vasc Interv Radiol 2010;21:224–230.
95 Moreno-Luna LE, Yang JD, Sanchez W, et al: Efficacy and safety of transarterial radioembolization versus chemoembolization in patients with hepatocellular carcinoma. Cardiovasc Intervent Radiol 2012;DOI: 10.1007/s00270-012-0481-2.
96 D'Avola D, Inarrairaegui M, Bilbao JI, et al: A retrospective comparative analysis of the effect of Y90-radioembolization on the survival of patients with unresectable hepatocellular carcinoma. Hepatogastroenterology 2009;56:1683–1688.
97 Bruix J, Raoul JL, Sherman M, et al: Efficacy and safety of sorafenib in patients with advanced hepatocellular carcinoma: subanalyses of a phase III trial. J Hepatol 2012;57:821–829.
98 Sato K, Lewandowski RJ, Bui JT, et al: Treatment of unresectable primary and metastatic liver cancer with yttrium-90 microspheres (TheraSphere): assessment of hepatic arterial embolization. Cardiovasc Intervent Radiol 2006;29:522–529.
99 Bilbao JI, de Martino A, de Luis E, et al: Biocompatibility, inflammatory response, and recanalization characteristics of nonradioactive resin microspheres: histological findings. Cardiovasc Intervent Radiol 2009;32:727–736.
100 Cheng AL, Kang YK, Chen Z, et al: Efficacy and safety of sorafenib in patients in the Asia-Pacific region with advanced hepatocellular carcinoma: a phase III randomized, double-blind, placebo-controlled trial. Lancet Oncol 2009;10:25–34.
101 Woodall CE, Scoggins CR, Ellis SF, et al: Is selective internal radioembolization safe and effective for patients with inoperable hepatocellular carcinoma and venous thrombosis? J Am Coll Surg 2009;208:375–382.
102 Uchino K, Tateishi R, Shiina S, et al: Hepatocellular carcinoma with extrahepatic metastasis: clinical features and prognostic factors. Cancer 2011;117:4475–4483.
103 Leung TW, Lau WY, Ho SK, et al: Radiation pneumonitis after selective internal radiation treatment with intraarterial 90yttrium-microspheres for inoperable hepatic tumors. Int J Radiat Oncol Biol Phys 1995;33:919–924.
104 Carr BI: Hepatic arterial 90Yttrium glass microspheres (Therasphere) for unresectable hepatocellular carcinoma: interim safety and survival data on 65 patients. Liver Transpl 2004;10:S107–S110.
105 Carretero C, Munoz-Navas M, Betes M, et al: Gastroduodenal injury after radioembolization of hepatic tumors. Am J Gastroenterol 2007;102: 1216–1220.
106 Riaz A, Gates VL, Atassi B, et al: Radiation segmentectomy: a novel approach to increase safety and efficacy of radioembolization. Int J Radiat Oncol Biol Phys 2011;79:163–171.
107 Sangro B, Gil-Alzugaray B, Rodriguez J, et al: Liver disease induced by radioembolization of liver tumors. Cancer 2008;112:1538–1546.
108 Gil-Alzugaray B, Chopitea A, Iñarrairaegui M, et al: Prognostic factors and prevention of radioembolization-induced liver disease. Hepatology 2012;DOI: 10.1002/hep.26191.

Viszeralmedizin
Gastrointestinal Medicine and Surgery

Übersichtsarbeit · Review Article

Viszeralmedizin 2013;29:103–111
DOI: 10.1159/000351120

Online publiziert: 12. April 2013

Resektion und Lebertransplantation bei hepatozellulärem Karzinom

Stefan A. Farkas Hans Jürgen Schlitt

Klinik und Poliklinik für Chirurgie, Universtätsklinik Regensburg, Deutschland

Schlüsselwörter
Hepatozelluläres Karzinom · Leber · Leberresektion · Zirrhose · Lebertransplantation

Zusammenfassung

Hintergrund: Kurative Therapieverfahren für das hepatozelluläre Karzinom (HCC) sind die Resektion und die Lebertransplantation. Grundlage für die Therapieentscheidung ist bisher die Klassifikation der Barcelona Clinic Liver Cancer Group (BCLC). **Methode:** Basis dieser Arbeit ist eine selektive Literaturübersicht zur Therapie des HCC. Leitlinien verschiedener Fachgesellschaften wurden einbezogen und aktuelle Arbeiten zu neuen chirurgischen Techniken besonders berücksichtigt. **Ergebnisse:** Primär resektable HCCs sollen reseziert werden. Für die Resektion kommen alle Patienten in adäquatem Allgemeinzustand ohne Zirrhose oder mit Child-A-Zirrhose ohne ausgeprägte portale Hypertension in Betracht. Hierbei ist von entscheidender Bedeutung, dass über die Möglichkeit der Resektabilität in einem ausgewiesenen Leberzentrum befunden wird. Auf die Leber beschränkte Rezidive können erneut operiert oder für eine Lebertransplantation gelistet werden. Techniken zur erweiterten Leberresektion und laparoskopische Verfahren finden zunehmend Anwendung und müssen weiter evaluiert werden. **Schlussfolgerung:** Neben der Resektion ist die Lebertransplantation inzwischen eine Standardtherapie für HCCs in Zirrhose. Innerhalb der Mailand-Kriterien können nach der Transplantation 5-Jahres-Überlebensraten von 70–90% erreicht werden. Allerdings erfordern der zunehmende Organmangel und die daraus resultierenden längeren Wartezeiten mit der Gefahr des Tumorprogresses ein Umdenken. So können Patienten, die für eine Transplantation infragekommen, nicht nur zum Bridging bis zur Transplantation reseziert werden, sondern auch, um eine biologische Stratifizierung durchzuführen. Unter engmaschigem Monitoring kann dann erst bei Auftreten eines Rezidivs eine «Rescue»-Transplantation durchgeführt werden. Jedoch werden auch Patienten mit fortgeschritteneren Tumoren, die nicht oder erst zu spät transplantiert werden können, zunehmend mit guten Ergebnissen reseziert. Somit könnten die Kriterien für eine Resektion im Rahmen der BCLC-Klassifikation erweitert werden.

Keywords
Hepatocellular carcinoma · Liver · Liver resection · Cirrhosis · Liver transplantation

Summary

Resection and Liver Transplantation of Hepatocellular Carcinoma

Background: Curative strategies for hepatocellular carcinoma (HCC) are liver resection and transplantation. The Barcelona Clinic Liver Cancer Group (BCLC) classification is the basis for therapeutic stratification. **Method:** This overview is based on a selective literature search on therapeutic strategies for HCC. Guidelines of different societies were taken into account while new surgical approaches were especially evaluated. **Results:** Primary resectable HCCs should be resected. Most patients without cirrhosis qualify for resection. A liver resection should be considered for patients with Child A cirrhosis but without severe portal hypertension and a stable health status. It is of utmost importance that resectability is evaluated in a designated liver center. Intrahepatic tumor recurrences can also be re-resected or listed for liver transplantation. New techniques for extended liver resections or minimally invasive liver resections are commonly used and need to be studied further. **Conclusion:** In addition to liver resection, liver transplantation represents a standard therapy for HCC in cirrhosis today. Whilst observing selection criteria, 5-year survival rates of 70–90% can be achieved. However, increasing organ shortage leads to longer waiting times and thus to a higher risk of tumor progress. Thus, if possible, patients eligible for transplantation could be primarily resected as a bridging therapy as well as biological stratification. Liver transplantation should then be offered as a 'rescue transplantation' if recurrence under close monitoring occurs. However, even patients with tumors in an advanced stage for which transplantation is not possible or too late can be resected with encouraging results. Therefore, the resection criteria according to the BCLC classification could be extended.

KARGER

Fax +49 761 4 52 07 14
Information@Karger.com
www.karger.com

1662-6664/13/0292-0103$38.00/0

Accessible online at:
www.karger.com/vim

PD Dr. Stefan A. Farkas, MBA
Klinik und Poliklinik für Chirurgie
Universitätsklinikum Regensburg
Franz-Josef-Strauß-Allee 11, 93053 Regensburg, Deutschland
stefan.farkas@ukr.de

Einführung

Die Therapie des hepatozellulären Karzinoms (HCC) orientiert sich heute im Großen und Ganzen an der «Barcelona Clinic Liver Cancer Group (BCLC)»-Klassifikation, die das Ausmaß des Tumors, den Grad der Zirrhose (Child-Stadium) und auch den klinischen Zustand des Patienten berücksichtigt [1]. Einzig aus der BCLC-Klassifikation lassen sich direkt therapeutische Konsequenzen ableiten (Abb. 1). Prinzipiell stehen drei kurative Therapieverfahren zur Behandlung des HCC zur Verfügung: die chirurgische Resektion, die orthotope Lebertransplantation sowie die Tumorablation. In Abhängigkeit von der Größe, Lage und Anzahl der Tumoren, der Leberrestfunktion bzw. dem Allgemeinzustand und gegebenenfalls Komorbiditäten soll im Rahmen einer interdisziplinären Konferenz die individuelle Therapie festgelegt werden. Von entscheidender Bedeutung ist hierbei, dass die Möglichkeit der Resektabilität in einem Leberzentrum von einem erfahrenen Leberchirurgen evaluiert wird.

Für die Resektion kommen prinzipiell alle Patienten ohne Zirrhose und Patienten in adäquatem Allgemeinzustand mit Child-A-Zirrhose ohne wesentliche portale Hypertension in Betracht (BCLC-Stadium 0) [1, 2].

Hepatozelluläres Karzinom ohne Zirrhose

Primär resektable HCCs sollen reseziert werden [3–5]. Große Fortschritte und die Standardisierung in der Leberchirurgie in den letzten zwei Jahrzehnten haben dazu geführt, dass bei gesunder Leber Resektionsausmaße von bis zu 80% mit geringer Morbidität und Mortalität erreicht werden können.

Kriterien der Nichtresektabilität sind die nichtresektable extrahepatische Tumormanifestation, die allgemeine Inoperabilität aufgrund der Komorbidität des Patienten sowie die fehlende funktionelle Reserve [4]. Insbesondere die Größe des Tumors alleine ist nur in Ausnahmefällen ein Ausschlusskriterium; entscheidend ist die Lage des Tumors in Bezug zu den Gefäßen. Aber auch eine Infiltration von Lebervenen ist kein alleiniges Ausschlusskriterium, da diese rekonstruiert werden können. Besonders bei großen Tumoren können gut atypische Resektionen durchgeführt werden; hierbei wird möglichst viel Lebergewebe belassen und der Patient verliert nur wenig funktionelles Lebergewebe. In nichtzirrhotischen Lebern ist ein funktionelles Residualvolumen von 25% ausreichend; d.h., es können bis zu 75% einer gesunden Leber reseziert werden. Hierbei ist zu berücksichtigen, dass das HCC selbst meist nicht mehr zur Funktion der Leber beiträgt und somit bei der Berechnung des notwendigen funktionellen Residualvolumens vernachlässigt werden kann. Deshalb ist von entscheidender Bedeutung, dass die Beurteilung der chirurgischen Resektabilität durch einen in der hepatobiliären Chirurgie erfahrenen Chirurgen im Rahmen einer interdisziplinären Konferenz erfolgt. Potenziell resektable Tumoren können bei Primärdiagnose aufgrund eingeschränkter funktioneller Reserve oder nicht möglicher R0-Resektion gegebenenfalls neoadjuvant behandelt werden (transarterielle Chemoembolisation, TACE). Hierfür eignet sich auch die operative Hypertrophieinduktion durch «in-situ splitting» mit Pfortaderligatur.

Bei nichtzirrhotischen Lebern beträgt die 5-Jahres-Überlebensrate allerdings nur 40–60%, da hier meist eine aggressivere Tumorbiologie vorliegt. Prognostische Faktoren für ein Rezidiv in nichtzirrhotischen Lebern sind der Residualtumorstatus, die Gefäßinvasion und das Tumorgrading [6–8].

Fibrolamelläres Karzinom

Das fibrolamelläre Karzinom ist eine seltene Sonderform des HCC ohne zugrunde liegende Zirrhose oder Hepatitis mit besonderen pathologischen Merkmalen und aggressiver Tumorbiologie, die typischerweise bei jungen Patienten auftritt (Abb. 2, 3). Die wenigen publizierten Daten zeigen ein 5-Jahres-Überleben von 37–76%. Allerdings liegt das rekurrenzfreie 5-Jahres-Überleben nur bei 18%. Lymphknotenmetastasen sind ein negativer prognostischer Faktor. Das mediane

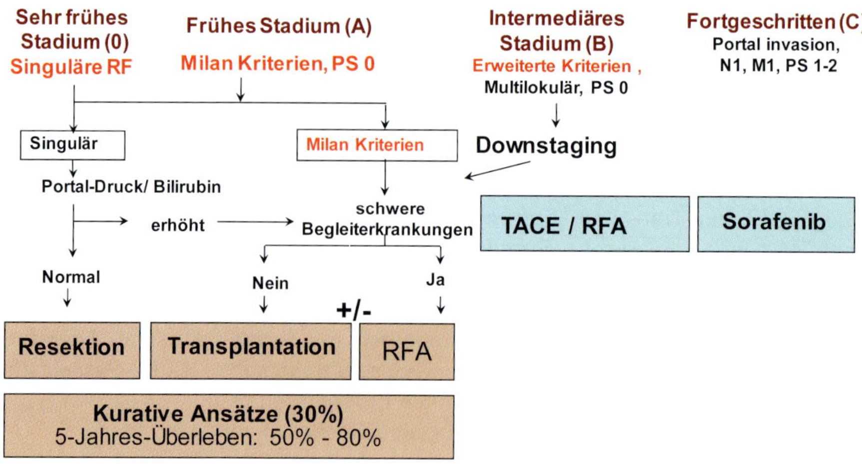

Abb. 1. Behandlungsstrategie von HCCs (modifiziert nach BCLC) (PS = Performancestatus).

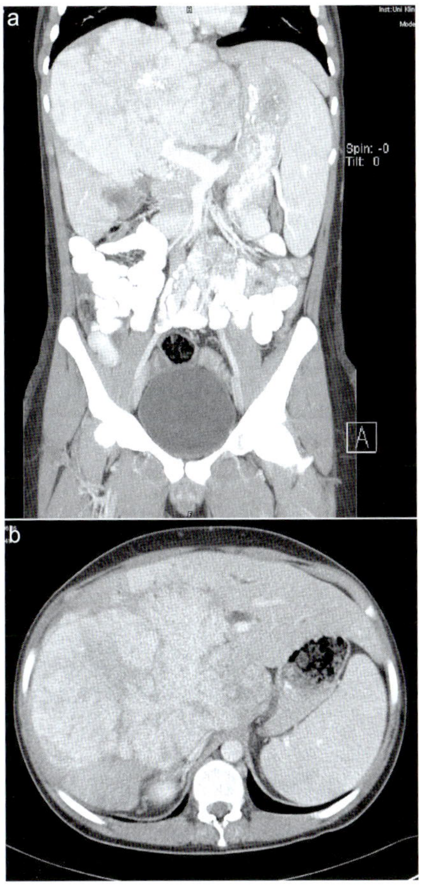

Abb. 2.a,b. Großes fibrolamelläres Karzinom bei einem 18-jährigen Patienten.

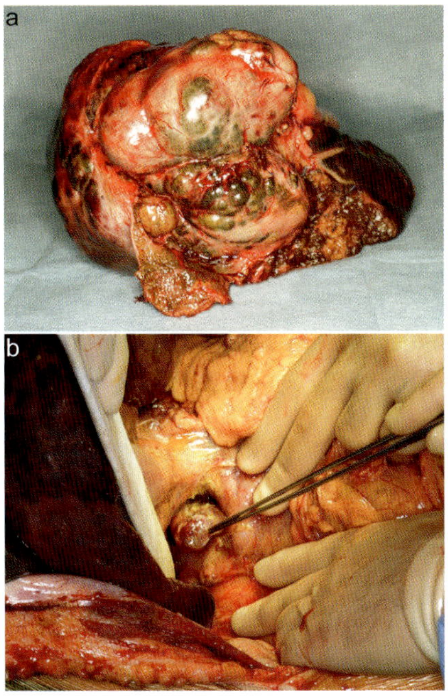

Abb. 3.a. Resektionspräparat. **b** Lymphknotendissektion im Hilus.

Überleben ohne Resektion liegt bei 12 Monaten [9]. Da späte Rezidive häufig sind, sollten auch Re-Resektionen durchgeführt und gegebenenfalls – bei fehlendem Lymphknotenbefall – auch eine Transplantation erwogen werden, da keine anderen effektiven Therapiestrategien für das fibrolamelläre Karzinom bestehen [10].

Leberresektion in Zirrhose

Die Resektion eines HCC in Zirrhose setzt eine sorgfältige Patientenevaluation voraus. Für die Resektion des HCC kommen Patienten in gutem klinischem Allgemeinzustand mit Child-A-Zirrhose in Betracht (BCLC-Stadium 0) [3–5].

In Einzelfällen können auch Patienten mit Child-B-Zirrhose reseziert werden. Das Vorliegen einer portalen Hypertension (Aszites, Thrombozyten <100 000, Splenomegalie) ist kein alleiniges Ausschlusskriterium für die Resektion, erhöht jedoch das operative Risiko. Hierbei muss im Hinblick auf das Ausmaß der portalen Hypertension im Einzelfall eine Nutzen-Risiko-Analyse der Resektion als alleiniger kurativer Therapieansatz durchgeführt werden. Im Zweifelsfall kann hierfür eine explorative Laparoskopie zur makroskopischen Beurteilung der Leber hilfreich sein. Insbesondere das präoperative Vorhandensein von Aszites weist jedoch auf einen protrahierten und somit komplizierteren postoperativen Verlauf hin.

Die funktionelle Resektabilität soll die ausreichende postoperative Leberfunktion und die portale Hypertension berücksichtigen. Bei einer Child-A-Zirrhose werden mehr als 40% des Leberparenchyms benötigt. Verschiedene Verfahren zur Evaluation der Leberfunktion über das Child-Pugh-System hinaus – wie der Indocyanin-Grün-Test oder der Limax-Test – sind entwickelt worden, konnten sich aber bisher in der Routine noch nicht durchsetzen. Um möglichst parenchymsparend zu operieren, ist die Durchführung nichtanatomischer Resektionen sinnvoll, da sich kein Unterschied bezüglich der Rezidivhäufigkeit gezeigt hat. Letztendlich ist für die Resektabilität die Einschätzung eines erfahrenen Leberchirurgen in enger Absprache mit dem Hepatologen entscheidend.

Notwendigkeit der optimierten Bildgebung zur Operationsplanung

Zur Planung der operativen Therapie ist eine optimierte Bildgebung notwendig. Standard ist – über das CT-Thorax/-Abdomen zum Staging hinaus – ein 3-Phasen-CT der Leber. Weiterhin ist als komplementäre Bildgebung eine dynamische Magnetresonanztomographie der Leber mit leberspezifischem Kontrastmittel sinnvoll. Der Ultraschall bzw. kontrastmittelverstärkte Ultraschall (contrast-enhanced ultrasound, CEUS) soll komplementär durchgeführt werden [11]. Darüber hinaus dient eine Fluor-18-Fluorodesoxyglukose-Positronenemissionstomografie (FDG-PET) sowohl zur Detektion extrahepatischer Metastasen als auch zur prognostischen Evaluation des HCC, da es den Differenzierungsgrad des HCC reflektiert [12, 13]. Leider ist das PET bei eher gut differenzierten und kleinen HCCs negativ, sodass es als Screening-Methode ungeeignet ist.

Intraoperativer Ultraschall ist Standard

Ein intraoperativer Ultraschall (IOUS) ist unbedingt notwendig, um weitere Herde zu detektieren und um die Operationsstrategie optimal festlegen zu können. An unserem Zentrum haben wir insbesondere sehr gute Erfahrungen mit intraoperativem kontrastmittelgestütztem Ultraschall (intraoperativer CEUS) mit linearer Sonde gemacht. Hiermit konnten wir intraoperativ 50% mehr Herde als im alleinigen B-Bild finden [14, 15]. Diese Methode wird derzeit weiter evaluiert.

Großer Sicherheitsabstand zum Tumor nicht unbedingt notwendig

Bei einer potenziell kurativen Resektion des HCC hat der früher geforderte weite Sicherheitsabstand von 2 cm in Studien keinen Vorteil bezüglich eines lokalen Rezidivs gezeigt [16]. Allerdings konnte in einer anderen Studie speziell bei kleineren Tumoren (HCC < 2 cm) gezeigt werden, dass der größere Sicherheitsabstand vor allem auch beim Vorliegen von Mikrometastasen einen Überlebensvorteil bringt [17]. Ursächlich für diese unterschiedlichen Ergebnisse ist möglicherweise eine unterschiedliche Tumorbiologie, da langsam wachsende große Tumoren oft ein weniger aggressives Wachstum haben als kleinere Tumoren mit Satellitenherden oder Mikrometastasen. Ein weiterer «Sicherheitsabstand» zur Resektionsfläche kann auch durch zusätzliche intraoperative Thermoablation erreicht werden. Eine zu erwartende R1-Situation hiernach ist somit keine Kontraindikation für eine Resektion. Daher sind speziell bei größeren Tumoren auch erweiterte Resektionen mit nur geringem Abstand oder gegebenenfalls auch mit einer R1-Situation hin zu einer zu erhaltenden Lebervene sinnvoll.

Erneute Resektion von auf die Leber beschränkten Rezidiven

Auch Re-Resektionen bei Rezidiven sind sinnvoll, da hier ebenfalls, insbesondere bei nicht extrahepatischem Tumorwachstum, 5-Jahres-Überlebensraten von bis zu 80% erreicht werden können. Diesbezüglich konnte in einer großen multivariaten Analyse gezeigt werden, dass die Re-Resektion die Therapie der Wahl bei Patienten ist, bei denen primär ein Herd reseziert wurde, die ein Jahr lang rezidivfrei waren und die keine portale Infiltration zeigen [18].

Ergebnisse nach Resektion von solitären oder kleinen HCCs in Zirrhose

Die besten Ergebnisse finden sich nach der Resektion von kleinen und solitären HCC-Herden in Zirrhose. In selektionierten Patientengruppen kann hiermit ein 5-Jahres-Überleben von 30–50% erreicht werden [19–21]. In einer aktuellen japanischen Registeranalyse [2] mit mehr als 20 000 Patienten lag das rezidivfreie 10-Jahres-Überleben bei 22%. Hierbei zeigten sich die Tumorgröße (>5 cm) und die Differenzierung als prognosebestimmend [2]. In anderen Studien gelten neben der Tumorgröße ein Alpha-Fetoprotein (AFP) > 1000 µg/l, das Vorliegen einer R1-Situation nach Resektion sowie eine mikrovaskuläre Infiltration als Risikofaktoren für ein Tumorrezidiv [22, 23]. Da unter anderem die mikrovaskuläre Infiltration nicht präoperativ bestimmt werden kann, sind hier neue diagnostische Tools notwendig, um eine bessere Prognose- und somit Therapiebestimmung durchführen zu können. Das FDG-PET ist in diesem Zusammenhang ein möglicher Ansatz [13].

Leberresektion versus Radiofrequenzablation in Zirrhose

Entsprechend der aktuellen Datenlage kann keine eindeutige Aussage zugunsten der Resektion oder Radiofrequenzablation (RFA) getroffen werden. Beide Methoden sind zur Therapie kleiner HCCs (<5 cm) in zirrhotischen Lebern akzeptabel. Eine aktuelle Metaanalyse zeigt, dass die Resektion im Vergleich zur RFA mit signifikant besserem Gesamt- und rezidivfreiem Überleben assoziiert ist. Allerdings findet sich nach einer Resektion auch eine signifikant höhere Komplikationsrate. Bei HCC-Herden >3 cm sollte der RFA eine Embolisation vorgeschaltet werden. Aufgrund des Risikos einer peritonealen Tumoraussaat bei subkapsulär gelegenen HCCs ist hier die Operation vorteilhaft. Zentrale kleine Läsionen in Zirrhose sind hingegen teilweise einfacher mittels RFA zu therapieren.

Neue chirurgische Techniken für erweiterte oder weniger invasive Leberresektionen

Erweitertes Leberresektionsverfahren «in-situ split»: Pfortaderligatur und Parenchymdurchtrennung zur schnellen Hypertrophieinduktion

Bis dato standen verschiedene Methoden zur Verfügung, um aus nichtresektablen resektable Tumoren zu machen. Zum einen gibt es die Möglichkeit der zweizeitigen Resektion bei multifokalen Tumoren. Hierbei wird zunächst der Tumor in einem Leberlappen reseziert und anschließend nach entsprechender Regeneration die zweite Seite operativ angegangen. Eine andere Möglichkeit ist die radiologische Pfortaderembolisation oder die operative Pfortaderligatur der tumortragenden Leberseite, sodass die kontralaterale Seite an Volumen und funktionalem Gewebe zunehmen kann. Auf diese Weise erreicht man eine Hypertrophie von etwa 10–46% in einem Zeitraum von 2–8 Wochen und eine Resektabilität von 70–100% in ausgewählten Fällen [24, 25]. Problematisch ist allerdings, dass bis zu 40% der Patienten aufgrund des langen Zeitraums zwischen Pfortaderembolisation und Resektion einen Tumorprogress zeigen, der einen kurativen Ansatz bzw. eine Resektion verhindert.

Am Universitätsklinikum Regensburg wurde, gemeinsam mit anderen Universitätskliniken, nun ein neues Verfahren evaluiert, bei dem die Pfortaderligatur mit einer kompletten Parenchymdissektion entlang des Ligamentum falciforme hepatis kombiniert wird (sogenanntes «in-situ split»). Hierbei wurde bei den 25 ausgewerteten Patienten vor der Komplettierungsoperation nach 9 Tagen eine mediane Volumenzunahme des linkslateralen Segments von 310 auf 536 ml gemessen. Dies entspricht im Median einem Anstieg um 74%. Die Überlebensrate im Gesamtkollektiv betrug nach einjähriger Follow-up-Periode 83% [26]. Diese Technik wurde nun durch andere Zentren bestätigt und findet mittlerweile in einigen Leberzentren Anwendung [27, 28], dies auch in Kombination mit laparoskopischer Resektionstechnik [29]. Die langfristigen Ergebnisse müssen weiter evaluiert werden.

Laparoskopische Leberresektion

Laparoskopische Leberresektionen finden zunehmend bei ausgewählten Patienten Anwendung. Hierbei werden rein laparoskopische, laparoskopisch assistierte und handassistierte Techniken voneinander unterschieden. Mit allen drei Methoden können in erfahrenen Leberzentren mit entsprechender laparoskopischer Expertise gute onkologische Langzeitergebnisse erreicht werden. Allerdings existiert eine deutliche Lernkurve für größere laparoskopische Leberresektionen.

Beim laparoskopischen Vorgehen besteht nicht nur ein kosmetischer Vorteil, sondern vor allem Patienten mit Zirrhose können von dem kleineren Zugangsweg profitieren. Dies gilt insbesondere für die postoperative Aszitesbildung mit konsekutiver Fasziendehiszenz, die bei Child-A-Zirrhose auch ohne portale Hypertension häufiger auftritt. Darüber hinaus können auch notwendige Rezidiveingriffe aufgrund der geringeren Verwachsungen möglicherweise leichter durchgeführt werden. Dies trifft auch für Patienten zu, die nach Resektion aufgrund eines Rezidivs innerhalb der Mailand-Kriterien transplantiert werden müssen. In einer aktuellen Studie fand sich bei Patienten, die nach initial laparoskopischer Leberresektion wegen eines Rezidivs transplantiert werden mussten, eine geringere Operationszeit und ein geringerer Blutverlust.

In einer aktuellen Metaanalyse wurden 29 Fallserien mit insgesamt mehr als 2600 Patienten untersucht [30]. Hierbei handelte es sich um selektionierte Patienten zumeist ohne Zirrhose, bei denen sich ähnliche Ergebnisse wie nach konventioneller Resektion zeigten. Die spezifische Erfahrung des Chirurgen beeinflusste die Ergebnisse deutlich, sodass eine Lernphase als notwendig angesehen wird. Die handassistierte und laparoskopisch assistierte Technik war mit einem besseren perioperativen Outcome assoziiert. Von den drei oben beschriebenen Techniken sollte somit die rein laparoskopische Technik dem erfahrenen Chirurgen vorbehalten sein. Die laparoskopisch assistierte Technik wurde vor allem in zirrhotischen Lebern, bei Tumoren mit ungünstiger Lokalisation und bei der Leber-Lebendspende verwendet.

Daten zum langfristigen onkologischen Outcome liegen nur in wenigen Studien vor. Hierzu hat die Gruppe um Cherqui Ergebnisse von drei europäischen Zentren zu Patienten mit HCC zusammengefasst [31]. In einer prospektiven Datenanalyse wurden 163 laparoskopische Leberresektionen untersucht. Von diesen Patienten hatten 120 (73%) eine Zirrhose. Bei 95% der Patienten wurde ein rein laparoskopisches Vorgehen gewählt. Die mediane Tumorgröße lag bei 3,7 cm. Es zeigte sich auch hier, dass nach einer gewissen Lernkurve die Komplikationen geringer und das Langzeitüberleben besser waren. In der aktuelleren Patientengruppe betrug das Gesamtüberleben nach 1, 3 und 5 Jahren jeweils 92,6, 68,7 und 64,9%, und das rezidivfreie Überleben belief sich auf 77,5, 47,1 bzw. 32,2%.

In einer aktuellen Zentrumsanalyse wurden das offene und das laparoskopische Vorgehen zumeist bei Patienten mit Zirrhose verglichen. Hier zeigten sich – allerdings bei kleiner Fallzahl – ein geringerer Blutverlust, weniger Komplikationen und ein kürzerer Krankenhausaufenthalt bei gleichem Langzeitüberleben [32].

Allerdings gibt es Grenzen für laparoskopische Resektionen. Dies sind vor allem Tumoren in den kranial gelegenen Lebersegmenten IVa, VII und VIII. Darüber hinaus sind große, sehr hilusnah gelegene oder an die Vena cava heranreichende Tumoren für das laproskopische Vorgehen weniger geeignet.

Weitere Studien werden die Komplikationen, das Langzeitüberleben und die ökonomischen Faktoren (längere Operationszeiten und teureres Equipment) in größeren Patientenkollektiven erfassen müssen.

Lebertransplantation für hepatozelluläres Karzinom in Zirrhose

Gesichertes HCC in Zirrhose innerhalb der «Mailand-Kriterien» als Indikation für Lebertransplantation

Basierend auf internationalen Studiendaten ist die Lebertransplantation bei der Anwendung von restriktiven Kriterien mit 5-Jahres-Überlebensraten von 70% assoziiert [33–35]. Darüber hinaus wird auch die zugrunde liegende Zirrhose behoben, die ebenfalls für die Entstehung des Tumors verantwortlich ist und zudem ein eigenes Mortalitätsrisiko mit sich bringt. Für die Transplantation geeignet sind unter anderem Patienten, die primär aufgrund eines Child-Stadiums B–C oder einer ausgeprägten portalen Hypertension nicht reseziert werden können (BCLC-Stadium A–C). Der Mangel an postmortalen Organspendern macht jedoch eine Selektion der Patienten hinsichtlich ihres Überlebens notwendig. Bei Vorliegen von extrahepatischer Tumormanifestation oder makroskopischer Gefäßinvasion ist eine Lebertransplantation kontraindiziert [3–5].

Die besten Prädiktoren für das Überleben von Patienten mit HCC nach Lebertransplantation sind die Mailand-Kriterien [33–37]. Patienten, die die Mailand-Kriterien (ein Knoten <5 cm oder bis zu 3 Knoten <3 cm, Abwesenheit von makro-

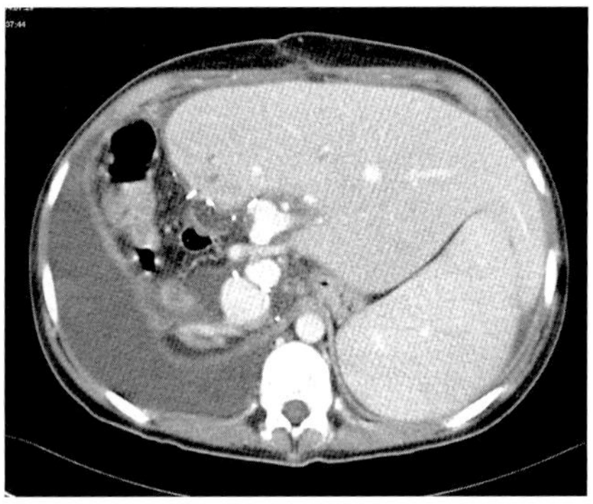

Abb. 4. Wochen nach erweiterter Leberresektion mit Gefäßrekonstruktion.

vaskulärer Infiltration) (Abb. 4) erfüllen und keine extrahepatischen Metastasen aufweisen, können im Eurotransplant-Bereich für eine Lebertransplantation gelistet werden. Sie erhalten hierfür eine standardisierte, akzeptierte Sonderregelung. Hierbei muss der Tumor durch mindestens eine der drei folgenden Methoden nachgewiesen werden:

- Biopsie;
- AFP > 400 und Hypervaskularisation in *einer* Bildgebung;
- Hypervaskularisation in *zwei* Bildgebungsverfahren.

Diese so selektionierten Patienten erreichen 5-Jahres-Überlebensraten von bis zu 70% und eine Lokalrezidivrate von unter 15%. Patienten außerhalb der Mailand-Kriterien können zwar gelistet werden, erhalten die Sonderregelung für HCC jedoch nicht. Weitere prognostische Kriterien sind die sogenannten UCSF(University of California San Francisco)-Kriterien. Diese fordern eine Tumorgröße <6,5 cm bei einem solitären Herd, weniger als 3 HCC-Herde mit einem Maximaldurchmesser des größten Herdes von <4,5 cm oder eine maximale Summe der addierten Tumordurchmesser <8 cm. Auch mit diesen Kriterien kann eine 5-Jahres-Überlebensrate von bis zu 70% erreicht werden [38]. Damit ist die Überlebenswahrscheinlichkeit der Patienten nach Transplantation ungefähr mit derjenigen von Patienten vergleichbar, die an einer Leberzirrhose ohne HCC leiden.

Sonderregelung für Patienten mit HCC innerhalb der Mailand-Kriterien

Die Kriterien für HCC-Patienten zur Transplantation sind aktuell im deutschen Transplantationsgesetz und bei der Allokation durch Eurotransplant verbindlich verankert. HCC-Patienten innerhalb der Mailand-Kriterien erhalten dabei eine standardisierte, akzeptierte Sonderregelung, die zu einem sukzessiven Punktgewinn und somit de facto einem Vorrücken auf der Warteliste auch bei stabiler Organfunktion führt. Ansonsten werden Lebern im Eurotransplant-Bereich nach dem MELD-System (Model for End-Stage Liver Disease; kalkulierter Wert aus Kreatinin, Bilirubin und International Normalized Ratio) alloziert. Somit konnte ein HCC-Patient mit stabiler Organfunktion mit einer Wartezeit von nur ungefähr einem Jahr rechnen. Allerdings hat sich aufgrund der dramatischen Verschlechterung der Organspendesituation in den letzten Jahren besonders in Deutschland die Wartezeit für diese Patienten deutlich verlängert. Außerdem wurden aufgrund der Möglichkeit der Sonderregelung auch mehr Patienten mit HCC für die Lebertransplantation gelistet, was wiederum zu einer Zunahme des Organmangels führt.

Downstaging, Tumorkontrolle und «Bridging» bis zur Lebertransplantation durch Resektion, TACE und RFA

Bei Patienten mit nichtresektablem HCC und bestehender Indikation zur Transplantation, aber fehlendem adäquatem Spenderorgan stellt die Wartezeit vor der Lebertransplantation ein hohes Risiko dar, aufgrund von Tumorprogression aus den engen Transplantationskriterien, die für Tumorgröße und -anzahl gelten, herauszufallen (Drop-out) [39]. Für das HCC innerhalb der Mailand-Kriterien korreliert daher die Drop-out-Rate mit der Länge der Wartezeit und der Größe des Tumors. Bei Patienten mit 2–3 HCC-Herden oder einem singulären HCC >3 cm berichten Yao et al. [38] über Drop-out-Raten nach 6, 12 und 18 Monaten von 12, 56 und 89% gegenüber solchen von 0, 10 und 21% bei einem singulären HCC <3 cm. Zum Überbrücken (Bridging) der Wartezeit – und mit dem Ziel, den Tumor innerhalb der Transplantationskriterien zu halten – haben sich in den letzten Jahren ablative Verfahren (RFA) sowie die TACE etabliert. Sie haben den Vorteil einer geringen Invasivität, gelten als sicher sowie parenchymschonend und sind mehrfach wiederholbar. Patienten mit HCC auf der Warteliste müssen alle 3 Monate mit einem schnittbildgebenden Verfahren bezüglich des Tumorprogresses kontrolliert werden. Hierbei wird zum einen die Wirksamkeit der Bridging-Verfahren und zum anderen ein Progress des Tumors untersucht. Wenn der nicht kontrollierbare Tumorprogress einen Drop-out aus den Mailand-Kriterien bedingt, muss der Patient von der Warteliste genommen werden. Somit werden Patienten mit einer aggressiveren Tumorbiologie, die nach einer Transplantation auch ein deutlich schlechteres Überleben als die anderen Patienten hätten, tumorbiologisch selektioniert.

Leber-Lebendspende als Option

Durch eine Leber-Lebendspende lässt sich die Wartezeit vermeiden und damit der mögliche Tumorprogress verhindern. Darüber hinaus entlastet dies den limitierten Pool an postmortalen Spenderorganen. Da das potenzielle Komplikationsrisiko für den Spender in erfahrenen Zentren relativ gering ist, sollte diese Möglichkeit bei Vorhandensein eines geeigneten Spenders evaluiert werden. Die Komplikationen und das Überleben nach Lebendspende sind für den Empfänger mit der postmortalen Spende vergleichbar. Allerdings kann die Lebendspende – im Gegensatz zur postmortalen Spende

– beim klinisch stabilen Patienten zum optimalen Zeitpunkt erfolgen und bietet daher einen entscheidenden Vorteil gegenüber der postmortalen Spende (Abb. 4).

Rezidivrisiko und Nachsorge

Nach einer Lebertransplantation wird durch die notwendige lebenslange Immunsuppression mit Calcineurininhibitoren das Rezidivrisiko erhöht. Die Ergebnisse der multinationalen Silver-Studie mit mTOR-Inhibitor als antitumoröser Immunsuppression sind abzuwarten [40, 41].

Patienten mit HCC und Lebertransplantation müssen engmaschig (im ersten Jahr alle 3 Monate, dann jährlich) mittels Bildgebung und AFP nachgesorgt werden.

Primäre Transplantation versus primäre Leberresektion und Transplantation als «Rescue»-Therapie

Wie bereits beschrieben, ist die Lebertransplantation theoretisch die beste Therapie für HCCs innerhalb der Mailand-Kriterien. Allerdings ist die Verfügbarkeit von postmortalen Organen limitiert und das Risiko eines Tumorprogresses aufgrund der längeren Wartezeiten nicht unerheblich. Besonders in Deutschland ist der Organmangel eklatant.

Eine mögliche Resektion des Tumors bei Patienten mit Child-A-Zirrhose als initiale Therapie vor der Listung zur Lebertransplantation hat folgende Vorteile: Zum einen kann diese als primäre Therapieoption unabhängig von der Zirrhose fungieren; zum anderen können durch die vollständige histologische Aufarbeitung eine Gefäßinvasion und Mikrosatellitenherde detektiert werden. Dies dient wiederum der Selektion der Patienten auf der Warteliste. Darüber hinaus ist die Resektion sofort verfügbar und bietet eine optimale Tumorkontrolle [42]. Die Resektion des HCC vor der Lebertransplantation dient somit nicht nur zur Kontrolle des Tumorwachstums sowie der Gefäßinvasion während der Wartezeit und damit dem Verbleib auf der Warteliste, sondern auch der tumorbiologischen Selektion der Patienten.

Cherqui et al. [43] untersuchten 67 Patienten mit HCC in Zirrhose innerhalb der Mailand-Kriterien, die primär leberreseziert wurden, anstatt für eine Transplantation gelistet zu werden. Die postoperative Morbidität betrug 34% und die Mortalität 4,5%. Nach einem mittleren Follow-up von 4,8 Jahren hatten 54% der Patienten ein intrahepatisches Rezidiv. Von diesen Patienten wurden wiederum 44% transplantiert, wenn sie die Altersgrenze nicht überschritten und das Rezidiv innerhalb der Mailand-Kriterien war. Das Gesamt- und das rezidivfreie Überleben in diesem Patientenkollektiv betrug 72 und 44%. Somit konnte trotz der signifikanten Rezidivrate mit einem engmaschigen postoperativen Monitoring eine sogenannte «Rescue»-Transplantation bei 61% der Patienten immer noch durchgeführt werden. Dadurch stehen mehr Organe für andere Patienten zur Lebertransplantation zur Verfügung. Um dieses pragmatische und organsparende Vorgehen zu belegen, muss allerdings eine randomisierte kontrollierte Studie durchgeführt werden.

Leberresektion als definitive Therapie

Eine Transplantation kommt jedoch für ältere Patienten (>75 Jahre) auch als «Rescue»-Therapie nicht infrage. Und auch jüngere Patienten mit HCC außerhalb der Mailand-Kriterien, die somit nicht unter eine Sonderregelung fallen, warten zu lange auf eine Transplantation. Somit muss die Leberresektion als definitive Therapie zunehmend in Betracht gezogen werden. Dies gilt auch für Patienten mit HCC innerhalb der Mailand-Kriterien, die aber auch aufgrund des Organmangels so lange warten, dass das Risiko eines Tumorprogresses während der Wartezeit weiter zunimmt. Resektionen werden deshalb auch zunehmend bei fortgeschrittenen Tumoren (BCLC-Stadium B und C) durchgeführt [44, 45]. Torzilli et al. [44] konnten zeigen, dass bei sorgfältiger Patientenselektion und adäquater parenchymsparender chirurgischer Technik unter Anwendung des IOUS große Tumoren mit vaskulärer Infiltration sowie niedriger Morbidität und Mortalität reseziert werden können [44]. Das Gesamtüberleben der 28 Patienten im BCLC-Stadium C nach der Resektion betrug nach 3 Jahren 70%, das rezidivfreie Überleben allerdings nur 34%. Auch andere aktuelle Beobachtungsstudien konnten zeigen, dass die über die letzten Dekaden deutlich besser werdenden Langzeitergebnisse der Leberresektion inzwischen bezüglich des Gesamtüberlebens mit der Lebertransplantation vergleichbar sind [45–48]. Dies wurde sowohl für Patienten mit HCC innerhalb der Mailand-Kriterien [47] als auch für HCC außerhalb der Mailand-Kriterien [45] gezeigt, gilt allerdings nur für das Gesamtüberleben und nicht für das rezidivfreie Überleben [35]. Zur Verbesserung des Gesamtüberlebens benötigen die Patienten eine lebenslange engmaschige postoperative Nachsorge mit optimierter Schnittbildgebung und sofortiger Therapie des Rezidivs [46]. Effektivere lokal ablative Verfahren als Alternative zur Re-Resektion sind hierfür notwendig.

Zusammenfassend lässt sich sagen, dass eine Erweiterung bzw. Revision der BCLC-Kriterien hin zur Resektion auch in fortgeschritteneren Stadien für einige Patientengruppen sinnvoll erscheint. Hierfür ist die Durchführung einer prospektiven Studie notwendig.

Disclosure Statement

HJS hat Vortragshonorare und Reisekostenerstattung von Novartis, Astellas, Pfizer und Roche erhalten. Er erfährt Forschungsunterstützung durch Pfizer und Novartis.

SAF erhielt Vortragshonorare und Reisenkostenerstattung bzw. bekommt Forschungsunterstützung von Novartis, Astellas, Roche und Pfizer.

Literatur

1 Bruix J, Llovet JM: Prognostic prediction and treatment strategy in hepatocellular carcinoma. Hepatology 2002;35:519–524.

2 Eguchi S, Kanematsu T, Arii S, Omata M, Kudo M, Sakamoto M, Takayasu K, Makuuchi M, Matsuyama Y, Monden M: Recurrence-free survival more than 10 years after liver resection for hepatocellular carcinoma. Br J Surg 2011;98:552–557.

3 Makuuchi M, Kokudo N, Arii S, Futagawa S, Kaneko S, Kawasaki S, Matsuyama Y, Okazaki M, Okita K, Omata M, Saida Y, Takayama T, Yamaoka Y: Development of evidence-based clinical guidelines for the diagnosis and treatment of hepatocellular carcinoma in Japan. Hepatol Res 2008;38:37–51.

4 Benson AB III, Abrams TA, Ben-Josef E, et al: NCCN clinical practice guidelines in oncology: hepatobiliary cancers. J Natl Compr Canc Netw 2009;7:350–391.

5 Poon D, Anderson BO, Chen LT, Tanaka K, Lau WY, Van CE, Singh H, Chow WC, Ooi LL, Chow P, Khin MW, Koo WH: Management of hepatocellular carcinoma in Asia: consensus statement from the Asian Oncology Summit 2009. Lancet Oncol 2009;10:1111–1118.

6 Lang H, Sotiropoulos GC, Brokalaki EI, Schmitz KJ, Bertona C, Meyer G, Frilling A, Paul A, Malago M, Broelsch CE: Survival and recurrence rates after resection for hepatocellular carcinoma in noncirrhotic livers. J Am Coll Surg 2007;205: 27–36.

7 Laurent C, Blanc JF, Nobili S, Sa CA, le Bail B, Bioulac-Sage P, Balabaud C, Capdepont M, Saric J: Prognostic factors and longterm survival after hepatic resection for hepatocellular carcinoma originating from noncirrhotic liver. J Am Coll Surg 2005;201:656–662.

8 Dupont-Bierre E, Compagnon P, Raoul JL, Fayet G, de Lajarte-Thirouard AS, Boudjema K: Resection of hepatocellular carcinoma in noncirrhotic liver: analysis of risk factors for survival. J Am Coll Surg 2005;201:663–670.

9 Stipa F, Yoon SS, Liau KH, Fong Y, Jarnagin WR, D'Angelica M, Abou-Alfa G, Blumgart LH, DeMatteo RP: Outcome of patients with fibrolamellar hepatocellular carcinoma. Cancer 2006;106:1331–1338.

10 Schlitt HJ, Neipp M, Weimann A, Oldhafer KJ, Schmoll E, Boeker K, Nashan B, Kubicka S, Maschek H, Tusch G, Raab R, Ringe B, Manns MP, Pichlmayr R: Recurrence patterns of hepatocellular and fibrolamellar carcinoma after liver transplantation. J Clin Oncol 1999;17:324–331.

11 McWilliams JP, Yamamoto S, Raman SS, Loh CT, Lee EW, Liu DM, Kee ST: Percutaneous ablation of hepatocellular carcinoma: current status. J Vasc Interv Radiol 2010;21(suppl 8):S204–S213.

12 Sorensen M, Frisch K, Bender D, Keiding S: The potential use of 2-[^{18}F]fluoro-2-deoxy-D-galactose as a PET/CT tracer for detection of hepatocellular carcinoma. Eur J Nucl Med Mol Imaging 2011;38: 1723–1731.

13 Seo S, Hatano E, Higashi T, Hara T, Tada M, Tamaki N, Iwaisako K, Ikai I, Uemoto S: Fluorine-18 fluorodeoxyglucose positron emission tomography predicts tumor differentiation, P-glycoprotein expression, and outcome after resection in hepatocellular carcinoma. Clin Cancer Res 2007;13(Pt 1): 427–433.

14 Loss M, Schneider J, Uller W, Wiggermann P, Scherer MN, Jung W, Schlitt HJ, Stroszczynski C, Jung EM: Intraoperative high resolution linear contrast enhanced ultrasound (IOUS) for detection of microvascularization of malignant liver lesions before surgery or radiofrequeny ablation. Clin Hemorheol Microcirc 2012;50:65–77.

15 Loss M, Jung EM, Scherer MN, Farkas SA, Schlitt HJ: Chirurgische Therapie von Lebermetastasen. Chirurg 2010;81:533–541.

16 Poon RT, Fan ST, Ng IO, Wong J: Significance of resection margin in hepatectomy for hepatocellular carcinoma: a critical reappraisal. Ann Surg 2000; 231:544–551.

17 Shi M, Guo RP, Lin XJ, Zhang YQ, Chen MS, Zhang CQ, Lau WY, Li JQ: Partial hepatectomy with wide versus narrow resection margin for solitary hepatocellular carcinoma: a prospective randomized trial. Ann Surg 2007;245:36–43.

18 Minagawa M, Makuuchi M, Takayama T, Kokudo N: Selection criteria for repeat hepatectomy in patients with recurrent hepatocellular carcinoma. Ann Surg 2003;238:703–710.

19 Fong Y, Sun RL, Jarnagin W, Blumgart LH: An analysis of 412 cases of hepatocellular carcinoma at a Western center. Ann Surg 1999;229:790–799.

20 Gouillat C, Manganas D, Saguier G, Duque-Campos R, Berard P: Resection of hepatocellular carcinoma in cirrhotic patients: longterm results of a prospective study. J Am Coll Surg 1999;189:282–290.

21 Lang H, Broelsch CE: Resektion und Transplantation bei Lebertumoren. Internist (Berl) 2007;48: 30–39.

22 Kim BW, Kim YB, Wang HJ, Kim MW: Risk factors for immediate post-operative fatal recurrence after curative resection of hepatocellular carcinoma. World J Gastroenterol 2006;12:99–104.

23 Shah SA, Greig PD, Gallinger S, Cattral MS, Dixon E, Kim RD, Taylor BR, Grant DR, Vollmer CM: Factors associated with early recurrence after resection for hepatocellular carcinoma and outcomes. J Am Coll Surg 2006;202:275–283.

24 Liu H, Zhu S: Present status and future perspectives of preoperative portal vein embolization. Am J Surg 2009;197:686–690.

25 Abulkhir A, Limongelli P, Healey AJ, Damrah O, Tait P, Jackson J, Habib N, Jiao LR: Preoperative portal vein embolization for major liver resection: a meta-analysis. Ann Surg 2008;247:49–57.

26 Schnitzbauer AA, Lang SA, Goessmann H, Nadalin S, Baumgart J, Farkas SA, Fichtner-Feigl S, Lorf T, Goralcyk A, Horbelt R, Kroemer A, Loss M, Rummele P, Scherer MN, Padberg W, Konigsrainer A, Lang H, Obed A, Schlitt HJ: Right portal vein ligation combined with in situ splitting induces rapid left lateral liver lobe hypertrophy enabling 2-staged extended right hepatic resection in small-for-size settings. Ann Surg 2012;255:405–414.

27 Aloia TA, Vauthey JN: Associating liver partition and portal vein ligation for staged hepatectomy (ALPPS): what is gained and what is lost? Ann Surg 2012;256:e9.

28 Sala S, Ardiles V, Ulla M, Alvarez F, Pekolj J, de Santibañes E: Our initial experience with ALPPS technique: encouraging results. Updates Surg 2012; 64:167–172.

29 Conrad C, Shivathirthan N, Camerlo A, Strauss C, Gayet B: Laparoscopic portal vein ligation with in situ liver split for failed portal vein embolization. Ann Surg 2012;256:e14–e15.

30 Lin NC, Nitta H, Wakabayashi G: Laparoscopic major hepatectomy: a systematic literature review and comparison of 3 techniques. Ann Surg 2013; 257:205–213.

31 Dagher I, Belli G, Fantini C, Laurent A, Tayar C, Lainas P, Tranchart H, Franco D, Cherqui D: Laparoscopic hepatectomy for hepatocellular carcinoma: a European experience. J Am Coll Surg 2010;211:16–23.

32 Cheung TT, Poon RT, Yuen WK, Chok KS, Jenkins CR, Chan SC, Fan ST, Lo CM: Long-term survival analysis of pure laparoscopic versus open hepatectomy for hepatocellular carcinoma in patients with cirrhosis: a single-center experience. Ann Surg 2013;257:506–511.

33 Mazzaferro V, Regalia E, Doci R, Andreola S, Pulvirenti A, Bozzetti F, Montalto F, Ammatuna M, Morabito A, Gennari L: Liver transplantation for the treatment of small hepatocellular carcinomas in patients with cirrhosis. N Engl J Med 1996;334: 693–699.

34 Mazzaferro V, Chun YS, Poon RT, Schwartz ME, Yao FY, Marsh JW, Bhoori S, Lee SG: Liver transplantation for hepatocellular carcinoma. Ann Surg Oncol 2008;15:1001–1007.

35 Mazzaferro V, Llovet JM, Miceli R, et al: Predicting survival after liver transplantation in patients with hepatocellular carcinoma beyond the Milan criteria: a retrospective, exploratory analysis. Lancet Oncol 2009;10:35–43.

36 Jonas S, Bechstein WO, Steinmuller T, Herrmann M, Radke C, Berg T, Settmacher U, Neuhaus P: Vascular invasion and histopathologic grading determine outcome after liver transplantation for hepatocellular carcinoma in cirrhosis. Hepatology 2001;33:1080–1086.

37 Yi NJ, Suh KS, Kim T, Kim J, Shin WY, Lee KU: Current role of surgery in treatment of early stage hepatocellular carcinoma: resection versus liver transplantation. Oncology 2008;75(suppl 1):124–128.

38 Yao FY, Xiao L, Bass NM, Kerlan R, Ascher NL, Roberts JP: Liver transplantation for hepatocellular carcinoma: validation of the UCSF-expanded criteria based on preoperative imaging. Am J Transplant 2007;7:2587–2596.

39 Clavien PA, Lesurtel M, Bossuyt PM, Gores GJ, Langer B, Perrier A: Recommendations for liver transplantation for hepatocellular carcinoma: an international consensus conference report. Lancet Oncol 2012;13:e11–e22.

40 Schlitt HJ, Schnitzbauer AA: Hepatocellular carcinoma: agents and concepts for preventing recurrence after curative treatment. Liver Transpl 2011;17(suppl 3):S10–S12.

41 Schnitzbauer AA, Schlitt HJ, Geissler EK: Influence of immunosuppressive drugs on the recurrence of hepatocellular carcinoma after liver transplantation: a gap between basic science and clinical evidence. Transplantation 2011;91:1173–1176.

42 Belghiti J, Cortes A, Abdalla EK, Regimbeau JM, Prakash K, Durand F, Sommacale D, Dondero F, Lesurtel M, Sauvanet A, Farges O, Kianmanesh R: Resection prior to liver transplantation for hepatocellular carcinoma. Ann Surg 2003;238:885–892.

43 Cherqui D, Laurent A, Mocellin N, Tayar C, Luciani A, Van Nhieu JT, Decaens T, Hurtova M, Memeo R, Mallat A, Duvoux C: Liver resection for transplantable hepatocellular carcinoma: long-term survival and role of secondary liver transplantation. Ann Surg 2009;250:738–746.

44 Torzilli G, Donadon M, Marconi M, Palmisano A, Del Fabbro D, Spinelli A, Botea F, Montorsi M: Hepatectomy for stage B and C hepatocellular carcinoma in the Barcelona Clinic Liver Cancer classification: results of a prospective analysis. Arch Surg 2008;143:1082–1090.

45 Canter RJ, Patel SA, Kennedy T, D'Angelica MI, Jarnagin WR, Fong Y, Blumgart LH, Freeman RB, DeMatteo RP, Abt PL: Comparative analysis of outcome in patients with hepatocellular carcinoma exceeding the Milan criteria treated with liver transplantation versus partial hepatectomy. Am J Clin Oncol 2011;34:466–471.

46 Fan ST, Mau Lo C, Poon RT, Yeung C, Leung Liu C, Yuen WK, Ming Lam C, Ng KK, Ching Chan S: Continuous improvement of survival outcomes of resection of hepatocellular carcinoma: a 20-year experience. Ann Surg 2011;253:745–758.

47 Chua TC, Saxena A, Chu F, Morris DL: Hepatic resection for transplantable hepatocellular carcinoma for patients within Milan and UCSF criteria. Am J Clin Oncol 2012;35:141–145.

48 Facciuto ME, Rochon C, Pandey M, Rodriguez-Davalos M, Samaniego S, Wolf DC, Kim-Schluger L, Rozenblit G, Sheiner PA: Surgical dilemma: liver resection or liver transplantation for hepatocellular carcinoma and cirrhosis. Intention-to-treat analysis in patients within and outwith Milan criteria. HPB (Oxford) 2009;11:398–404.

Viszeralmedizin
Gastrointestinal Medicine and Surgery

Interdisziplinäres Gespräch · Interdisciplinary Discussion

Viszeralmedizin 2013;29:113–119
DOI: 10.1159/000350772

Online publiziert: 15. April 2013

Hepatozelluläres Karzinom – ein interdisziplinäres Krankheitsbild

Gesprächsleiter: Nisar Peter Malek (Tübingen) Ulf Peter Neumann (Aachen) Jens Ricke (Magdeburg)

Teilnehmer: Thomas Berg (Leipzig) Christiane Bruns (München) Timm Denecke (Berlin) Heinz-Josef Klumpen (Amsterdam) Hans Lippert (Magdeburg) Maciej Pech (Magdeburg) Markus Peck-Radosavljevic (Wien)

Frage 1: Die Erkennung und vor allem die Sicherung des hepatozellulären Karzinoms (HCC) bleiben kontrovers. Die maßgebenden Leitlinien erlauben den klinischen Beweis eines Karzinoms über nichtinvasive Bildgebung. Wie ist der Stellenwert der Leberbiopsie heute und zukünftig?

Denecke: Die relevantesten Therapieentscheidungen beim HCC, die von der Diagnosesicherung abhängen, sind die Resektion bzw. Lokalablation und die Lebertransplantation. Hierbei ist, neben der Kenntnis von Lage und Anzahl, die definitive und korrekte Identifizierung der Läsionen als HCC von sensibler Bedeutung. Bei der Gegenüberstellung der bildgebenden Diagnostik und der Biopsie steht die Sensitivität der Verfahren nicht zur Debatte, da nur biopsiert werden kann, was vorher durch die Bildgebung entdeckt wurde. Somit geht es hier um die Artdiagnose einer durch Bildgebung detektierten Läsion. Dabei ist der Verzicht auf eine Tumorbiopsie bei eindeutiger bildgebender Diagnostik von HCCs in Nachteilen der invasiven Biopsie und in der immer zuverlässigeren radiologisch-bildgebenden Diagnostik begründet.

Die Nachteile der perkutanen Biopsie bestehen zum einen in mehreren Risiken, wie z.B. der Blutung oder der Tumorzellverschleppung. Zum anderen ist der negativ prädiktive Wert der Biopsie, auch bei wiederholter Durchführung und trotz bildgeführter Technik, vor allem bei kleinen Tumoren eingeschränkt. Auch ist die feingewebliche Differenzialdiagnostik an Biopsiematerial, das nie die ganze Zielläsion repräsentiert, anspruchsvoll und führt nicht immer zur abschließend korrekten Diagnose. Aufgrund der Praktikabilität können auch nicht alle Kandidatläsionen eines Patienten auf bioptischem Wege gesichert werden.

Was die Läsionscharakterisierung in der radiologisch-bildgebenden Diagnostik angeht, so gelingt – selbst im kontrastmittelgestützten Ultraschall oder in der Computertomographie (CT) – mit relativ einfachen Kriterien für das Vorliegen eines HCC (d.h. arterielle Hyperkontrastierung und Auswaschphänomen in der Spätphase) in den meisten Fällen eine eindeutige Diagnose. Komplexer, aber bei guter Bildqualität der CT überlegen, ist die Läsionsbeurteilung in der Magnetresonanztomographie (MRT). Eine weitere Verbesserung der MRT-Diagnostik versprechen die hepatozytenspezifischen Kontrastmittel: Die späte Hepatozytenphase liefert einen zusätzlichen Parameter für die Detektion und Charakterisierung von potenziellen HCC-Manifestationen. Mit einer differenzialdiagnostischen Unsicherheit der Bildgebung muss vor allem dann gerechnet werden, wenn im Einzelfall eine technische oder patientenbedingte Einschränkung der Untersuchungsqualität besteht. Ist also die Biopsie von potenziellen HCC-Läsionen in Leitlinien durch die bildgebende Diagnostik generell ersetzt, so sollte auch eine konkrete Mindestanforderung an die Untersuchungstechnik und -qualität formuliert bzw. berücksichtigt werden. Zusammengenommen gelingt bei einem Großteil der potenziellen HCC-Läsionen anhand der radiologischen Diagnostik eine zuverlässige Artdiagnose mit geringer Fehlerquote. Dadurch können nach derzeit gängigen Kriterien in der Regel die möglichen Behandlungspfade korrekt gewählt werden, ohne dass eine Biopsie aktuell entscheidende weiterführende Erkenntnisse bringt. Bei nicht eindeutigem Bildbefund oder nicht ausreichend erzielbarer Bildqualität stellt die Biopsie jedoch eine hilfreiche Ergänzung dar.

Peck-Radosavljevic: Die aktuellen Leitlinien der Europäischen Lebergesellschaft (European Association for the Study of the Liver, EASL) zur Diagnostik und Therapie des HCC

KARGER
Fax +49 761 4 52 07 14
Information@Karger.com
www.karger.com

1662-6664/13/0292-0113$38.00/0

Accessible online at:
www.karger.com/vim

Prof. Dr. med. Jens Ricke
Klinik für Radiologie und Nuklearmedizin
Universitätsklinikum Magdeburg AöR
Leipziger Straße 44, 39120 Magdeburg, Deutschland
jens.ricke@med.ovgu.de

ermöglichen die nichtinvasive, rein radiologische Diagnosestellung eines HCC bei Läsionen über 1 cm Durchmesser und typischen Anfärbeverhalten in der mehrphasischen CT oder im dynamischen MRT. Der Kontrastmittelultraschall wird in diesen Leitlinien als unzureichend spezifisch nicht akzeptiert. Eine eindeutige Bildgebung ist in größeren Zentren zumindest bei der Hälfte bis zwei Dritteln der HCCs zu erwarten. In diesen Fällen ist die Durchführung einer minimal invasiven Biopsie zu rein diagnostischen Zwecken nicht notwendig. Das Hauptargument dagegen ergibt sich aus dem damit verbundenen Aufwand und dem diagnostischen Grundprinzip, dass Untersuchungen ohne therapierelevanten Mehrwert zu vermeiden sind, und weniger aus der Furcht vor Komplikationen, zumal die in der Literatur angegebenen Komplikationsraten sehr heterogen und in vielen Fällen überzeichnet sind. Klinisch relevante Blutungsepisoden sind bei radiologisch gezielten Biopsien eine Rarität, und über eine zweifelsfrei nachgewiesene und prognoserelevante, Biopsie-assoziierte Tumorzellverschleppung wurde bisher auch kaum berichtet.

Die wahre Stärke der Biopsie liegt jedoch nicht in der simplen Diagnosestellung, sondern in der bisher unersetzlichen Möglichkeit zur Materialgewinnung für eine molekularbiologische Charakterisierung des Tumors zur prognostischen Stratifizierung und gezielten Therapieentscheidung. Eine entsprechende nichtinvasive Tumordiagnostik ist heutzutage für das Mammakarzinom (Hormonrezeptorstatus, HER2/neu), für das Kolonkarzinom (kras-Mutationen) oder das Bronchialkarzinom nicht mehr vorstellbar. Für das HCC war das bis vor kurzer Zeit anders, da trotz erheblicher wissenschaftlicher Bemühungen bisher keine therapierelevante molekulare Klassifizierung des HCC gefunden werden konnte. Allerdings muss an dieser Stelle auch ganz klar festgestellt werden, dass gerade der unglückliche Umstand des häufig fehlenden bioptischen Materials in den letzten Jahren eine molekularbiologische Analyse und potenzielle Subgruppenidentifikation unmöglich gemacht hat. Als besonders bedauerliches Beispiel sei hier die Phase-III-Registrierungsstudie des Multikinaseinhibitors Sorafenib bei fortgeschrittenem HCC erwähnt, in der aufgrund des weitgehend fehlenden Biopsiematerials keine entsprechende Biomarkeranalyse durchgeführt werden konnte. Spätestens mit der Identifizierung des HGF(Hepatozyten-Wachstumsfaktor)-Rezeptors c-MET als eindeutigen prognostischen Faktor für Patienten mit HCC sowie dem klaren Überlebensvorteil durch den Einsatz des sich nun in Phase-III-Entwicklung befindlichen c-MET-Inhibitors Tivantinib wurde jedoch das Ende der nichtinvasiven Diagnostik eingeleitet, zumindest für die palliativen Stadien (BCLC-B, BCLC-C). Da gezielte Therapeutika wie Tivantinib nur in HCCs mit hoher Expression von c-MET im Tumorgewebe wirksam sind, ist für den Einsatz gezielter bzw. personalisierter Therapeutika eine Tumorbiopsie erlässlich. Mit der zu erwartenden Registrierung weiterer Therapeutika mit klarem molekularen Ansatzpunkt wird die Personalisierung auch in der Therapie des HCC deutlich zunehmen und eine bioptische Abklärung voraussetzen, obwohl die bekannten Schwächen der Biopsie wie Stichprobenfehler unwidersprochen sind. Die Fehler der letzten Jahre mit großzügiger, nichtinvasiver Diagnostik in mehreren gescheiterten großen Phase-III-Studien (Sunitinib, Brivanib, Erlotinib, Linifanib), die nun nicht einmal mehr nachträglich molekular für die Identifizierung von Biomarkern von Subgruppen mit einem potenziellen Behandlungsbenefit untersucht werden können, sind nicht mehr wiedergutzumachen und bedeuten schon jetzt einen unwiederbringlichen Wissensverlust über fast ein Jahrzehnt klinischer Hepatomforschung.

Auch wenn es aus radiologischer Sich in vielen Fällen leicht und eindeutig möglich ist, die Diagnose eines HCC nichtinvasiv zu stellen, so ist die minimal invasive gezielte Biopsie bereits heute und noch mehr für die Zukunft eine unverzichtbare Voraussetzung für das Management der Patienten und Patientinnen, für die eine aktive Therapie in Betracht kommt.

Frage 2: Entscheidend für die Prognose der Patienten mit HCC ist die Entdeckung in frühen Stadien. Der überwältigende Anteil der Patienten mit der Diagnose eines HCC in Deutschland wird mit weit fortgeschrittenen Tumoren vorstellig. Wie sieht ein vernünftiges Screening-Programm aus? Welches Vorgehen empfehlen Sie insbesondere niedergelassenen Kollegen und wie definieren Sie Risikopatienten?

Berg: Das HCC eignet sich in besonderer Weise für Früherkennungsstrategien, da die Risikopatienten für die HCC-Entwicklung gut charakterisiert sind und die Erkrankung im Frühstadium kurativ zu behandeln ist. Jedoch werden aktuell weniger als 30% der Patienten in einem HCC-Stadium diagnostiziert, in denen kurative Therapieoptionen zum Einsatz kommen können. Die Gründe für diesen Befund sind vielfältig. Offenbar stellt sich jedoch weniger die Frage, wie, sondern ob Screening- bzw. Surveillance-Untersuchungen bei Personen mit erhöhtem HCC-Risiko zum Einsatz kommen. Risikopatienten für die HCC-Entwicklung werden entweder nicht identifiziert oder nur zu einem geringen Anteil in Überwachungsuntersuchungen eingeschlossen. Nach Statistiken US-amerikanischer Krankenkassen wurden Patienten mit HCC im Vorfeld vor der Diagnosestellung zu nur ca. 40% von Gastroenterologen/Hepatologen betreut. Eine retrospektive Analyse aus Texas ergab, dass nur 20% aller Patienten, die sich mit der Diagnose eines HCC in einem Zentrum vorstellten, Screening-Untersuchungen erhalten hatten. Bei der Mehrzahl der Patienten war die chronische Lebererkrankung (20%) oder die Zirrhose (40%) nicht bekannt gewesen, oder es wurde kein Screening angeordnet (38%) bzw. nicht durchgeführt (3%). Wurden die Patienten von einem Hepatologen betreut, waren die Screening-Raten um das Sechsfache höher und bei Patienten mit Alkoholerkrankung um das Siebenfache geringer. Zu ähnlichen Ergebnissen kommt eine Studie der «National Veterans Administration» bei 1480 mit Hepatitis-C-Virus infizierten Patienten mit HCC. Der Prozentsatz der Patienten mit jährlichen Vorsorgeuntersuchungen (entweder Ultraschall oder Alpha-Fetoprotein (AFP)) betrug 34%. Eine jährliche Surveillance mit AFP und Sonographie bzw. sechsmonatige Intervalluntersuchungen mit mindestens einer Methode (Ultraschall oder AFP) erfolgte nur bei 2 bzw. 6% aller Patienten. Es ist durchaus wahrscheinlich, dass die US-amerikanischen Erfahrungen in gewissem Umfang auch auf die Situation in Deutschland übertragbar sind.

Die aktuellen europäischen und amerikanischen Leitlinien empfehlen alle 6 Monate die Durchführung von Früherkennungsuntersuchungen bei Patienten mit erhöhtem Risiko allein mittels Ultraschall. Die Serum-AFP-Konzentration als Baustein der nichtinvasiven HCC-Diagnostik wurde in den Leitlinienempfehlungen aufgrund der nur mäßigen Sensitivität und Spezifität dieses Markers aus dem diagnostischen Algorithmus herausgenommen. Prospektive Studien, die die Effektivität des HCC-Screenings bestätigten, haben jedoch sowohl Sonographie als auch AFP-Bestimmungen eingesetzt. Hohe oder im Verlauf langsam ansteigende AFP-Konzentrationen bei Patienten mit chronischen Lebererkrankungen bzw. Zirrhose (ohne aktuellen entzündlichen Schub) sind jedoch ein starkes Indiz für das Vorliegen eines HCC, sodass unter Berücksichtigung der Dynamik dieses Parameters die AFP-Bestimmung aus meiner Sicht weiterhin einen wertvollen Baustein in der Surveillance von Risikopatienten darstellt. Neue HCC-Serummarker wie Descarboxyprothrombin (DCP), glykosyliertes AFP (AFP-L3) oder Osteopontin werden allein oder in Kombination mit AFP evaluiert und könnten in Zukunft zu einer verbesserten Früherkennung des HCC beitragen.

Eine Verkürzung der Screening-Intervalle auf 3 Monate konnte nicht zu einer Steigerung der HCC-Früherkennungsrate beitragen. Auch bei engmaschigen Kontrolluntersuchungen mittels Ultraschall wird das HCC bei 20–30% aller Patienten erst in fortgeschrittenen Stadien (außerhalb der Milan-Kriterien) diagnostiziert. CT oder dynamisches MRT haben sich aufgrund der kostenintensiven Untersuchung sowie der Strahlenbelastung beim CT als Screening-Untersuchung nicht durchgesetzt. Sie sollten jedoch in Erwägung gezogen werden, wenn aufgrund von Adipositas, Darmgasüberlagerung oder anderen technischen Schwierigkeiten die Durchführung einer aussagekräftigen Ultraschalluntersuchung nicht möglich ist oder wenn sich ein kontinuierlicher Anstieg der AFP-Konzentrationen ohne sonographisches Korrelat zeigt.

Alle Patienten mit Leberzirrhose, unabhängig von der Genese der Erkrankung, bei denen potenziell Therapieoptionen bestehen, sollten HCC-Früherkennungsuntersuchungen erhalten. Die chronische Infektion mit dem Hepatitis-B-Virus (HBV) stellt unabhängig von einer Zirrhoseentstehung ein HCC-Risiko dar, sodass Patienten mit HBV-Infektion ebenfalls regelmäßig untersucht werden sollten.

Neuere epidemiologische Studien belegen auch für die nichtalkoholische Fettleberhepatitis (nonalcoholic steatohepatitis, NASH) ein signifikantes Risiko für die HCC-Entwicklung – und das auch bereits in präzirrhotischen Stadien. Liegt zusätzlich ein Diabetes mellitus vor, steigt das HCC-Risiko weiter an. Genetische Polymorphismen im «Patatin-like phospholipase domain containing 3»-Gen (PNPLA 3, Adiponutrin) sind vor allem bei nutritiv-toxischen Lebererkrankungen (alkoholische und nichtalkoholische Fettlebererkrankung) mit einem erhöhten HCC-Risiko assoziiert. Weitere Risikofaktoren für die HCC-Entwicklung auf dem Boden einer chronischen Lebererkrankung sind das männliche Geschlecht, hohes Alter, hoher Body-Mass-Index und ein Nikotinabusus. Anhand dieser Faktoren können Hochrisikopatienten für die HCC-Entwicklung definiert und risikoadaptierte Surveillance-Strategien etabliert werden.

Frage 3: Personalisierte Medizin ist ein Begriff, der viele Diskussionen in der Onkologie bestimmt und nicht nur von Ärzten oder Wissenschaftlern benutzt wird, sondern auch von Pharmakonzernen, Kostenträgern und der Politik. Was bedeutet personalisierte Medizin heute und morgen für das HCC – von der systemischen Therapie bis hin zur Ultima Ratio, der Transplantation? Welche Biomarker haben für Sie heute schon Relevanz?

Berg: Eine auf bestimmten molekularen Charakteristika des HCC basierende «personalisierte» HCC-Therapie – im klassischen Sinne einer personalisierten onkologischen Medizin – ist für das HCC nicht etabliert. Mit dem Multikinase-Inhibitor Sorafenib steht bisher nur eine zugelassene systemische Therapie zur Verfügung, die für alle Patienten mit fortgeschrittenem HCC bei noch ausreichender Leberfunktion empfohlen wird.

Zahlreiche Substanzen, die über zielgerichtete Angriffspunkte insbesondere die Proliferation und Angiogenese des HCC beeinflussen, befinden sich jedoch in der klinischen Entwicklung. Personalisierte Therapiestrategien in Abhängigkeit von molekularen Tumoreigenschaften werden daher in Zukunft mit hoher Wahrscheinlichkeit auch für Patienten mit HCC von Bedeutung sein. Beispiele hierfür stellen die zielgerichtete Therapie gegen Glypican-3 oder die MET-Rezeptor-Tyrosinkinase dar. Glypican-3 wird nur auf etwa 30% aller HCCs hochexprimiert und reguliert maßgeblich Prozesse des Zellwachstums sowie der Zelldifferenzierung und Migration. Die Effektivität eines rekombinanten humanisierten Antikörpers gegen Glypican-3 scheint nach ersten Analysen wesentlich vom Ausmaß der Glypican-3-Expression abhängig zu sein. Der Tyrosinkinase-Inhibitor Tivantinib führt nach Bindung an den MET-Rezeptor zu Apoptose und verminderter Proliferation und wird im Rahmen von Phase-III-Studien ausschließlich bei Patienten mit hoher MET-Expression evaluiert.

Stadium und Ätiopathogenese der chronischen Lebererkrankung, auf deren Boden das HCC entstanden ist, haben grundlegende Bedeutung für die Prognose und die Therapieoptionen der Tumorerkrankung. Genexpressionsprofile des den Tumor umgebenden Lebergewebes, nicht jedoch des Tumors selbst, zeigten eine signifikante Korrelation mit der Überlebenswahrscheinlichkeit. Die stadienabhängige Berücksichtigung molekularer Charakteristika der Lebererkrankung könnte somit einen weiteren wichtigen Aspekt im zukünftigen individualisierten Management des HCC darstellen, wird aber auch zu einer Steigerung der ohnehin hohen Komplexität personalisierter onkologischer Therapiekonzepte führen. Eine Sonderstellung im Kontext der personalisierten onkologischen Medizin besitzt das HCC auch dadurch, dass das therapeutische Armamentarium heterogen ist und sich die Relevanz potenzieller Biomarker in Abhängigkeit des Therapieverfahrens (resektiv, lokal ablativ oder systemisch) voneinander unterscheiden wird.

Die Therapie des HCC erfolgt unter Berücksichtigung des Tumorstadiums (insbesondere Zahl und Größe der HCC-Herde) und der Leberfunktion. Die Milan-Kriterien stellen den «benchmark» für die Auswahl von Patienten mit HCC für die Lebertransplantation dar. Die AFP-Konzentrationen erlauben darüber hinaus eine Einschätzung des individuellen HCC-Rezidivrisikos und werden bereits als «Biomarker» in Kombination mit den bildgebenden Kriterien für die Entscheidung zur Transplantation berücksichtigt. Wenngleich zahlreiche weitere Faktoren, z.B. das Grading oder der DNA-Index des Tumors, für die Prognoseabschätzung von Relevanz sind und Zahl und Größe nur in begrenztem Umfang die Biologie der Erkrankung reflektieren, hat sich noch kein anderer Marker für die Therapiestratifizierung etablieren können.

Personalisierte Therapiekonzepte sollten jedoch nicht ausschließlich auf eine immer feinere molekulare Charakterisierung der Tumor- bzw. Peri-Tumor-Erkrankung begrenzt werden, sondern sich aus der Synthese aller individuellen patientenbezogenen Befunde entwickeln. Sir William Osler (1849–1919) formulierte es folgendermaßen: «It is much more important to know what sort of a patient has a disease than what sort of a disease a patient has».

Bruns: Personalisierte Medizin bedeutet beim HCC ähnlich wie bei anderen Krebserkrankungen eine individuell auf das onkologische Risiko des jeweiligen Patienten «maßgeschneiderte» Therapie unter Berücksichtigung genereller Faktoren wie Alter des Patienten, Komorbiditätsprofil, Lebensqualität bis hin zu Patientenwunsch.

Die Lebertransplantation ist die onkologisch beste Therapie für das auf die Leber begrenzte HCC, da durch die Transplantation nicht nur die radikalste Resektion des Tumors, sondern auch zusätzlich die Entfernung des präneoplastischen Gewebes ermöglicht wird. Die Organverfügbarkeit sowie die aktuellen Allokationsrichtlinien (BCLC, AASLD oder EASL Guidelines) sind allerdings entscheidende Einflussgrößen der «maßgeschneiderten» Therapie für die Patienten, deren Erkrankungsstadium optimalerweise mit antizipiertem, bestmöglichem Langzeitergebnis durch Lebertransplantation behandelt werden könnten [1, 2]. Um während der entsprechend langen Wartezeit eine Tumorprogression zu vermeiden, erhalten diese Patienten eine neoadjuvante Überbrückungstherapie (Bridging). Hier steht eine Vielzahl von Bridging-Verfahren zur Verfügung, die stadienadaptiert, aber auch komplementär eingesetzt werden können. Lokoregionär ablative Verfahren (transarterielle Chemoembolisation, TACE), selektive interne Radiotherapie (SIRT), Radiofrequenzablation (RFA), stereotaktische Bestrahlung (Cyberknife), systemische Therapien mit dem Multityrosinkinase-Inhibitor Sorafenib oder auch die chirurgische Resektion können zur lokalen Tumorkontrolle während der Wartezeit eingesetzt werden und sind damit ein Teil des «maßgeschneiderten» Therapieansatzes beim HCC.

Die onkologische Wertigkeit aller neoadjuvanten Bridging-Ansätze ist bis dato nur unzureichend geklärt, insbesondere, ob sich dadurch die Tumorbiologie oder das Metastasierungsverhalten über den Zeitraum der Therapie oder nach Transplantation verändert. Entscheidend ist, dass i) dem Patient durch Ansprechen auf eine neoadjuvante Therapie der Zugang zur Lebertransplantation überhaupt ermöglicht wird und dass ii) Therapieansprechen als positiver Prognoseparameter bei günstiger Tumorbiologie gewertet wird. Im eigenen Krankengut korreliert das Überleben nach Transplantation mit dem Response-Grad nach RECIST. Demgegenüber wird zunehmend evidenter, dass die momentan basierend auf Tumorgröße und -anzahl geltenden Milan-Kriterien für den individuellen Patienten keine prognostische Wertung zulassen. Retrospektive Patientenanalysen legen nahe, dass HCCs, die durch neoadjuvante Therapien ein Downstaging innerhalb der Milan-Kriterien erfahren haben, eine ähnlich gute Prognose aufweisen wie Tumoren, die bei Diagnosestellung bereits innerhalb der Milan-Kriterien waren [3–5].

Weitere prädiktive oder prognostische Biomarker, die stadiengerechte, «maßgeschneiderte» Therapiekonzepte beim HCC relevant beeinflussen, gibt es bislang nicht.

Klumpen: Personalisierte Medizin ist das Zusammenspiel von Faktoren, die sich auf drei Hauptfaktoren beziehen: i) der Tumor, ii) der Patient, iii) die Behandlung. Bei der Aufklärung der ersten zwei Faktoren werden uns, neben retrospektiven Analysen, größere genetische Studien sicherlich weiterhelfen auf der Suche nach den richtigen Zielpunkten von Medikamenten und den Patienten, die den meisten Nutzen von einer Behandlung haben werden. Für den dritten Punkt will ich mich auf die medikamentöse Behandlung konzentrieren. Hierbei ist es wichtig zu wissen, dass ein Medikament neben dem richtigen Wirkungsmechanismus auch die richtige Dosis im Patienten erreichen muss, um optimal zu wirken. Für andere Medikamente sowie Antibiotika, Antidepressiva und Immunsuppressiva haben wir uns schon lange daran gewöhnt, dass dies wichtig ist, um einen bestimmten Blutspiegel zu erreichen. Das Einstellen auf den richtigen Blutspiegel erhöht den Nutzen der Behandlung und verhindert eine Über- oder Unterbehandlung, auch bei Krebsmedikamenten, und wird auch «therapeutic drug monitoring (TDM)» genannt [6]. Für das HCC und die Behandlung mit Sorafenib ist noch nicht deutlich, was der richtige Blutspiegel sein sollte, um eine Über- oder Unterbehandlung zu verhindern. Die empfohlene Dosis ist für alle Patienten die gleiche (2 × 400 mg pro Tag). Eine Anpassung dieser Dosis nach unten wird in der Praxis nur bei Unverträglichkeit angewandt. Eine Dosissteigerung bei dem Ausbleiben von Nebenwirkungen und fehlender Wirksamkeit ist nicht gebräuchlich, wäre jedoch logisch und sicherlich darin begründet, dass die Ausscheidung von Sorafenib im Laufe der Zeit zunimmt [7].

Für ein anderes Medikament, Imatinib, auch ein Tyrosinkinase-Inhibitor wie Sorafenib, sind die oben beschriebenen Phänomene bekannt, und es wird das Prinzip des TDM in der Klinik empfohlen [8, 9].

Genau wie bei Imatinib ist es auch bei Sorafenib so, dass eine große Inter-Patienten-Variabilität besteht, was den Blutspiegel bei gleicher Dosierung betrifft. Im Moment laufen verschiedene Studien, um den Zusammenhang zwischen dem Blutspiegel bei Sorafenib mit der Wirkung des Medikamentes zu korrelieren [10]. Komplizierend kommt hinzu, dass Sorafenib im Individuum in mehr oder weniger aktiven Metaboliten verschieden metabolisiert wird. Die Verteilung der Menge der Metaboliten ist von verschiedenen Faktoren abhängig, wie z.B. der Leberfunktion und der Komedikation. Es könnte also der Fall sein, dass nicht allein der Blutspiegel von Sorafenib selbst, sondern auch der Blutspiegel der Metaboliten wichtig ist, um die optimale Behandlung, also die personalisierte Medizin, zu erreichen. Davon ausgehend, dass wir innerhalb der nächsten Zeit wissen werden, bei welchem Tumor die besten Wirkungserfolge mit Sorafenib erzielt werden können und welchen Blutspiegel wir erreichen sollten, haben wir leider unser Ziel noch nicht erreicht. Es gibt noch das Problem der Verträglichkeit. Manche Patienten werden die Behandlung nicht vertragen, da ihr Metabolismus, möglicherweise genetisch bedingt, nicht die gewünschten Blutspiegel ohne unverträgliche Nebenwirkungen erreichen lässt.

Zusammenfassend sollte bei einer personalisierten Medizin neben der Individualisierung abhängig vom Tumor und den Patientenumständen auch die richtige Zieldosis bei der medikamentösen Behandlung bekannt sein. Die Resultate von laufenden Studien werden uns hierbei hoffentlich bald weiterhelfen.

Pech: Klassische Biomarker nutzen wir derzeit so gut wie nicht für die Indikationsstellung oder Durchführung einer interventionell-radiologischen Behandlung des HCC. Einen Stellenwert haben aber umgekehrt interventionelle Eingriffe als eigenständige Biomarker bzw. prognostische Faktoren.

Herr Professor Otto aus Mainz beispielsweise hat in früheren Arbeiten gezeigt, dass das Ansprechen auf eine Chemoembolisation als Bridging zur Transplantation sehr gut mit der Prognose der Patienten korreliert – Chemoembolisation dient hier also potenziell als Stratum für die Transplantationsindikation. Zukünftig von Wichtigkeit auch für minimal invasive Eingriffe könnte die Bestimmung von Serummarkern wie VEGF (vaskulärer endothelialer Wachstumsfaktor) oder anderen werden. Wir wissen mittlerweile, dass Bestrahlung oder Chemoembolisation der Leber angiogenetische Kaskaden eröffnen. VEGF hat in multiplen Studien einen negativen prognostischen Wert bewiesen. Derzeit ist nicht vorhersagbar, welcher Patient nach einer RFA, Bestrahlung oder Chemoembolisation einen VEGF-Anstieg erleidet; zukünftig wird es spannend sein, ob eine Unterbrechung der VEGF-Kaskaden oder anderer Angiogenese-Pfade durch spezifische Moleküle die Prognose der Patienten verbessert. Ansonsten verstehe ich den Begriff «personalisierte Medizin» eher als einen Vorgriff auf die Individualisierung der Therapiekonzepte und vor allem der Sequenzen des Werkzeugeinsatzes. Wir sehen sehr häufig, dass wir Patienten über Monate und Jahre mit unterschiedlichen Verfahren – sei es lokal, lokoregionär oder systemisch – behandeln, die sequenziell eingesetzt bzw. beim Restaging zum Follow-up nach beispielsweise 3 Monaten immer wieder neu entschieden werden. Ich glaube persönlich, dass die größten Prognosevorteile für das HCC auf dem Wege der perfekten Sequenzierung der Therapiemaßnahmen für individuelle Krankheitsentwicklungen zu erzielen sind.

Frage 4: Die Lebertransplantation ist die einzige definitive Therapie des HCC in Zirrhose. Wo sehen Sie die Lebertransplantation in zehn Jahren?

Bruns: Bislang gilt die Lebertransplantation als optimalste Therapie für Patienten mit hepatisch begrenzten HCCs. Diese Patienten erhalten zur Überbrückung der teilweise langen Wartezeit im Eurotransplant-Raum zur Verhinderung der Tumorprogression eine neoadjuvante Bridging-Therapie. Die jeweils beste Therapiemodalität wird bislang unter Berücksichtigung der Tumorlast, der Tumorlokalisation und des Allgemeinzustands des Patienten in einem interdisziplinären Tumorboard festgelegt.

Patienten mit Tumoren innerhalb der Milan-Kriterien werden Extrapunkte, d.h. Standard Exception (SE) Points, zugebilligt, wodurch in der Regel nach 12–18 Monaten über die reguläre Organvergabe eine Lebertransplantation ermöglicht wird. Ausgehend von einem initialen match-MELD (Model for End-Stage Liver Disease) von 22 Punkten, der einer 3-Monats-Mortalität von 15% entspricht, werden die Patienten alle 3 Monate um den Punktewert einer 3-Monats-Mortalität von 10% hochgestuft. Dabei ist bislang Folgendes zu berücksichtigen: i) Tumoren müssen vor der Listung je-derzeit innerhalb der Milan-Kriterien gelegen sein; ii) Tumoren, die nach Ansprechen auf eine neoadjuvante Bridging-Therapie die Milan-Kriterien erreichen, erhalten keine SE-Zusatzpunkte; iii) Tumoren müssen auch zum Zeitpunkt der Höherstufung in 3-Monats-Schritten immer die Milan-Kriterien erfüllen. Patienten mit Tumoren außerhalb der Milan-Kriterien erhalten selbst bei gutem Ansprechen auf eine neoadjuvante Therapie (auch bei Rückbildung bis innerhalb der Milan-Kriterien) keine Sonderpunkte und sind so trotz teilweise guter Prognose im Wesentlichen auf eine Leber-Lebendspende angewiesen.

Ein Fortschritt in der Lebertransplantation bei zugrunde liegendem HCC wäre einerseits die Weiterentwicklung in Richtung individualisierter, Biomarker-gestützter Bridging-Verfahren, um eine «maßgeschneiderte» neoadjuvante Therapie mit hoher Wahrscheinlichkeit einer Tumorresponse für jeden gelisteten Patienten zu erzielen.

Auch ist vorstellbar, dass die Response-Evaluation bei «maßgeschneiderter» neoadjuvanter Therapie zukünftig durch die Untersuchung molekularer Marker oder den Einsatz von molekularem Imaging verfeinert und wohlmöglich frühzeitiger erfassbar ist.

In ähnlicher Weise könnte ein Biomarker-unterstütztes onkologisches Risikoprofil unter Einbeziehung moderner Techniken zur Response-Evaluation und der Zeit der Krankheitsstabilität die bisherigen Allokationsrichtlinien zur Transplantation bei HCC ergänzen.

Es gibt bereits erste Initiativen in den USA und in Deutschland, Patienten mit nachgewiesener Tumorresponse auf neoadjuvante Therapien den Zugang zu einer Lebertransplantation im regulären Verteilungsverfahren zu erleichtern.

Berücksichtigt man die bleibende Organknappheit, ist ein Ausbau der Forschung im Bereich des «tissue engineerings» zur funktionellen Unterstützung marginaler Organangebote denkbar, wobei derartige Ansätze bei onkologischen Grunderkrankungen kritisch bleiben [11].

Lippert: Das HCC entsteht in der Zirrhose. Dies kann sowohl solitär als auch multilokulär sein. Hier lassen sich nur individuelle Konzepte umsetzen, die die Grunderkrankung, den Gesamtzustand und die lokale Situation einbeziehen. Mit einer Lebertransplantation wird das Organ mit dem Tumor entfernt. Dennoch werden Rezidive nach einer Lebertransplantation beschrieben. Die Milan-Kriterien sind heute die tragfähigste Entscheidungshilfe, weil sie Transplantationskandidaten potenziell auf heilbare, frühere Stadien reduzieren. Ich gehe davon aus, dass sich daran nichts ändern wird.

Schließt man die aktuellen Probleme der Transplantationsmedizin ein, so ist vor allem die kurzfristige Verfügbarkeit von Organen ein wesentlicher Faktor, der das Handeln bei frühen HCCs bestimmt. Das Bridging mittels Resektion, lokaler ablativer Therapie und einer Minderung der kanzerogenen Gefahr in der Zirrhoseleber ist mittlerweile und sicher auch weiterhin Standard.

Systematische Verbesserungen sind durch eine profunde medikamentöse Prophylaxe, individuelle Entscheidungen zu sparsamerer Resektion und hochpräzise Lokaltherapien im Sinne eines Downstagings über die nächsten 20 Jahre noch denkbar. Die Leber-Lebendspende kann die Organknappheit erheblich positiv beeinflussen. Keine höhere Effektivität durch eine Transplantation sehe ich bei cholangiozellulärem Karzinom.

Teilnehmer

Prof. Dr. med. Thomas Berg
Sektion Hepatologie, Department für Innere Medizin, Neurologie und Dermatologie
Medizinische Klinik und Poliklinik für Gastroenterologie und Rheumatologie
Universitätsklinikum Leipzig
Liebigstraße 20, 04103 Leipzig, Deutschland
thomas.berg@medizin.uni-leipzig.de

Prof. Dr. med. Christiane Bruns
Onkologische Chirurgie, Chirurgische Klinik und Poliklinik
Klinik für Allgemeine, Viszeral-, Transplantations-, Gefäß- und Thoraxchirurgie
LMU München – Campus Großhadern
Marchioninistraße 15, 81377 München, Deutschland
Christiane.Bruns@med.uni-muenchen.de

PD Dr. med. Timm Denecke
Klinik für Radiologie
Charité – Universitätsmedizin Berlin, Campus Virchow-Klinikum
Augustenburger Platz 1, 13353 Berlin, Deutschland
timm.denecke@charite.de

Dr. Heinz-Josef Klumpen
Medizinische Onkologie, Academisch Medisch Centrum
Universität von Amsterdam
Meibergdreef 9, 1105AZ Amsterdam, Niederlande
h.klumpen@amc.nl

Prof. Dr. med. Hans Lippert
Klinik für Allgemein-, Viszeral- und Gefäßchirurgie
Universitätsklinikum Magdeburg A.ö.R.
Leipziger Straße 44, Haus 10, 39120 Magdeburg, Deutschland
hans.lippert@med.ovgu.de

Prof. Dr. med. Maciej Pech
Klinik für Radiologie und Nuklearmedizin
Universitätsklinikum Magdeburg AöR
Leipziger Straße 44, 39120 Magdeburg, Deutschland
maciej.pech@med.ovgu.de

Ao. Univ. Prof. Dr. Markus Peck-Radosavljevic
Abteilung Gastroenterologie und Hepatologie
Medizinische Universität Wien
Währinger Gürtel 18–20, 1090 Wien, Österreich
markus.peck@meduniwien.ac.at

Literatur

1 European Association For The Study Of The Liver; European Organisation For Research And Treatment Of Cancer: EASL-EORTC clinical practice guidelines: management of hepatocellular carcinoma. J Hepatol 2012;56:908–943.
2 Bruix J, Sherman M: Management of hepatocellular carcinoma: an update. Hepatology 2011;53: 1020–1022.
3 Otto G, Herber S, Heise M, et al: Response to transarterial chemoembolization as a biological selection criterion for liver transplantation in hepatocellular carcinoma. Liver Transpl 2006;12: 1260–1267.
4 Ravaioli M, Grazi GL, Piscaglia F, et al: Liver transplantation for hepatocellular carcinoma: results of down-staging in patients initially outside the Milan selection criteria. Am J Transplant 2008; 8:2547–2557.
5 Yao FY, Kerlan RK Jr, Hirose R, et al: Excellent outcome following down-staging of hepatocellular carcinoma prior to liver transplantation: an intention-to-treat analysis. Hepatology 2008;48:819–827.
6 Gao B, Yeap S, Clements A, Balakrishnar B, Wong M, Gurney H: Evidence for therapeutic drug monitoring of targeted anticancer therapies. J Clin Oncol 2012;30:4017–4025.
7 Arrondeau J, Mir O, Boudou-Rouquette P, et al: Sorafenib exposure decreases over time in patients with hepatocellular carcinoma. Invest New Drugs 2012;30:2046–2049.
8 Teng JF, Mabasa VH, Ensom MH: The role of therapeutic drug monitoring of imatinib in patients with chronic myeloid leukemia and metastatic or unresectable gastrointestinal stromal tumors. Ther Drug Monit 2012;34:85–97.
9 Judson I: Therapeutic drug monitoring of imatinib – new data strengthen the case. Clin Cancer Res 2012;18:5517–5519.
10 Ricke J, Schuette K, Rosmorduc O, et al: Sorafenib in combination with local microtherapy guided by gadolinium-EOB-DTPA enhanced MRI in patients with inoperable hepatocellular carcinoma (HCC) (SORAMIC). ASCO Meeting Abstracts 2012;30(15s):TPS4148.
11 Török E, Lutgehetmann M, Bierwolf J, Melbeck S, Düllmann J, Nashan B, Ma PX, Pollok JM: Primary human hepatocytes on biodegradable poly(l-lactic acid) matrices: a promising model for improving transplantation efficiency with tissue engineering. Liver Transpl 2011;17:104–114.

Imprint

ISSN Print Edition: 1662–6664
ISSN Online Edition: 1662–6672

Journal Homepage: http://www.karger.com/vim

Publication Data: Volume 29, 2013 of 'Viszeralmedizin' appears with 6 issues.

Distribution and Subscription: Karger offers three types of subscription: Print Only, Online Only and the combined Print + Online. The basic annual subscription rate is the same for all three delivery forms; however, a fee for the combined print and online subscription is levied, and there is a postage and handling charge for Print Only and Print + Online. Subscriptions run for a full calendar year. Prices are given per volume.

Print subscription: EUR 197.– + postage and handling.
Online subscription: EUR 197.–.
Combined (print + online) subscription: EUR 247.– + postage and handling.

For customers in Germany: Please turn to your bookshop or to
S. Karger Verlag für Medizin und Naturwissenschaften GmbH
Wilhelmstr. 20A, 79098 Freiburg (Germany)
Tel. +49 761 45 20 70, Fax +49 761 45 20 714
E-mail information@karger.com

For customers in all other countries: Please contact your bookshop or
S. Karger AG, Allschwilerstr. 10, 4009 Basel (Switzerland)
Tel. +41 61 3 06 11 11, Fax +41 61 3 06 12 34
E-mail karger@karger.com

Advertising: Correspondence should be addressed to the publisher.
S. Karger Verlag für Medizin und Naturwissenschaften GmbH
Attn. Ellen Zimmermann (Head of Marketing)
E-mail e.zimmermann@karger.com

Price list No. 19 of January 1, 2013 is effective.

V.i.S.d.P. (Person responsible according to the German Press Law): Sibylle Gross

Type setting and printing: Kraft Druck GmbH, 76275 Ettlingen, Germany.

Bibliographic Services:
EMBASE / Excerpta Medica
Reference Update
Science Citation Index Expanded

KARGER

Fax +49 761 4 52 07 14
Information@Karger.com
www.karger.com

© 2013 S. Karger GmbH, Freiburg

Accessible online at:
www.karger.com/vim

Viszeralmedizin
Gastrointestinal Medicine and Surgery

Case Report · Fallbericht

Viszeralmedizin 2013;29:121–124
DOI: 10.1159/000350518

Online publiziert: 12. April 2013

Surgical Exploration as the Definitive Means of Diagnosing a Unilateral Idiopathic Retroperitoneal Fibrosis: Report of a Case

Achim Troja Nader El-Sourani Dalibur Antolovic Hans-Rudolph Raab

Department of General and Visceral Surgery, Oldenburg Hospital gGmbH, Germany

Keywords
Idiopathic retroperitoneal fibrosis · Ormond's disease

Summary
Background: Retroperitoneal fibrosis is considered as one of the rare diseases, with an incidence rate of 1/200,000. A guideline for its diagnosis and therapy does not exist. In the past centuries, case studies and small-scale series have therefore been used for diagnostic purposes. **Case Report:** We report the case of a 45-year-old female patient who approached the emergency department complaining of flank pain. The primary diagnostics including computed tomography, magnetic resonance imaging, sonography, and laboratory testing showed a distension of the Musculus psoas and Musculus iliacus on the right side with an unclear genesis. Accessorily performed diagnostic analysis including scintigraphy and intestinal endoscopy did not provide additional information. Because of persisting complaints, a surgical exploration of the right retroperitoneal space was performed resulting in a histological diagnosis of an idiopathic fibrosis (Morbus Ormond). **Conclusion:** Despite the permanent improvement of diagnostic imaging in general, a surgical exploration accompanied by histological investigation is the diagnostic tool of choice in selected cases.

Schlüsselwörter
Idiopathische retroperitioneale Fibrose · Morbus Ormond

Zusammenfassung
Hintergrund: Die retroperitoneale Fibrose wird mit einer Inzidenzrate von 1/200 000 als eine der seltenen Erkrankungen angesehen. Eine Richtlinie für deren Diagnose und Therapie ist nicht existent. In den vergangenen Jahrhunderten wurden daher Fallberichte und kleinere Studienserien zu diagnostischen Zwecken eingesetzt. **Fallbericht:** Wir berichten im Folgenden über eine 45-jährige Patientin, die sich mit Flankenschmerzen in unserer Notfallambulanz vorstellte. In der bildgebenden Diagnostik samt Computertomographie, Magnetresonanztomographie, Sonographie und laborchemischen Analysen zeigte sich eine Auftreibung unklarer Genese im Musculus psoas und Musculus iliacus. Ergänzende Endoskopien und eine durchgeführte Szintigraphie führten nicht zur Diagnosestellung. Bei persistierenden Beschwerden wurde anschließend eine retroperitoneale Exploration vorgenommen. Histologisch zeigte sich das Bild einer retroperitonealen Fibrose (Morbus Ormond). **Schlussfolgerung:** Trotz aller Verbesserungen in der bildgebenden Diagnostik stellt die chirurgische Exploration mit anschließender Histologie zeitweise das entscheidende Diagnostikum dar.

Introduction

Retroperitoneal fibrosis is considered as one of the rare diseases, with an incidence rate of 1/200,000. In the past centuries, case studies and small-scale series have been used for diagnostic purposes.

A guideline for its diagnosis and therapy does not exist. By means of a rare case study we would like to describe the complex procedure of diagnosing retroperitoneal fibrosis. In the following case study the improvement of medical imaging is not inevitably the key in making a diagnosis.

KARGER
Fax +49 761 4 52 07 14
Information@Karger.com
www.karger.com

1662-6664/13/0292-0121$38.00/0

Accessible online at:
www.karger.com/vim

Dr. Achim Troja
Klinik für Allgemein- und Viszeralchirurgie, Klinikum Oldenburg gGmbH
Rahel-Straus-Straße 10, 26133 Oldenburg, Germany
troja.achim@klinikum-oldenburg.de

Case Report

History

A 45-year-old female patient presented to the surgical emergency with diffuse, right-sided abdominal pain for 1 week. On admission, she described that the symptoms had started 1 week ago in her right flank, with a progression of pain over the last few days. The past medical history included an appendectomy 15 years ago and a reactive depression without pharmacological treatment.

On the day of presentation, we performed a computed tomography (CT) of the abdomen and the pelvis showing a diffuse swelling of the right psoas muscles with adjacent reaction of the retroperitoneum.

Findings

The clinical examination upon presentation showed tenderness in the right flank, right lumbar, and right iliac fossa. There were no other clinical findings. The laboratory results showed elevated inflammatory parameters (leukocytes 11,800/μl; C-reactive protein 9.0 mg/dl). All other values were within the normal range.

Considering the preliminary findings, the swelling of the psoas muscle in combination with the elevated inflammatory parameters suggested an inflammatory process. However, the CT and abdominal ultrasound could not diagnose the presence of a definitive abscess. The kidney was not involved in the inflammatory process, and the urine status did not show any abnormalities.

Further diagnostics included a magnetic resonance imaging (MRI) of the abdomen (fig. 1, 2). A distinct signal uptake was seen dorsal to the right kidney. The uptake stretched from the dorsal part of the right psoas muscle and the whole iliacus muscle, the autochthone back musculature, and into the subcutaneous tissue. The spinal cord, however, was normal. A definite focus could not be identified.

Therapy and Follow-up

Regarding the elevated inflammatory parameters in combination with the inflammatory changes of the right psoas and iliacus muscle seen in the imaging process, we started an antibiotic treatment with a third-generation cephalosporin and metronidazole due to the assumption of an underlying bacterial infection. Consultations in the department of urology and gynecology were without relevant findings. A bone scintigraphy was performed to exclude any ongoing inflammatory process of the spine. In order to eliminate an intestinal dignity, a colonoscopy as well as a MR Sellink was performed. Both investigations did not show any evidence for the above-described changes or a link to the inflammatory process.

The inflammatory parameters regressed under the antibiotic therapy; however, the subjective clinical signs persisted. Due to the unsatisfactory situation, a second MRI of the abdomen and pelvis was performed 14 days after antibiotic treatment and showed no relevant new findings. Since no focus could be identified, an open biopsy via a retroperitoneal approach was indicated. As no tumor was identified in the imaging procedures (CT and MRI), we decided to perform a small retroperitoneoscopy rather than a CT-guided probe.

Intraoperatively, we found a diffuse swelling of the muscle whereas the adjacent tissue was rather sclerotic/fibrotic. The histopathological assessment described an idiopathic retroperitoneal fibrosis, i.e. Ormond's disease. There was no sign of a malignant process. The postoperative period was without any complications. The patient was discharged a few days later for an outpatient follow-up.

Discussion

Although idiopathic retroperitoneal fibrosis was first described in 1905 by Albarran and was identified by J.K. Ormond as its own disease entity four decades later, Ormond's disease is considered a rare disease with an incidence rate of 1/200,000 [1, 2]. In 1948, Ormond first described two cases in which an inflammatory retroperitoneal mass was found in the presence of a ureter obstruction. In the following years, Ormond collected data of similar cases of unidentified ureter obstructions. He divided his collective data into two groups. The data of the first group described a symmetrical fibrosis whereas the second group described a localized process [3].

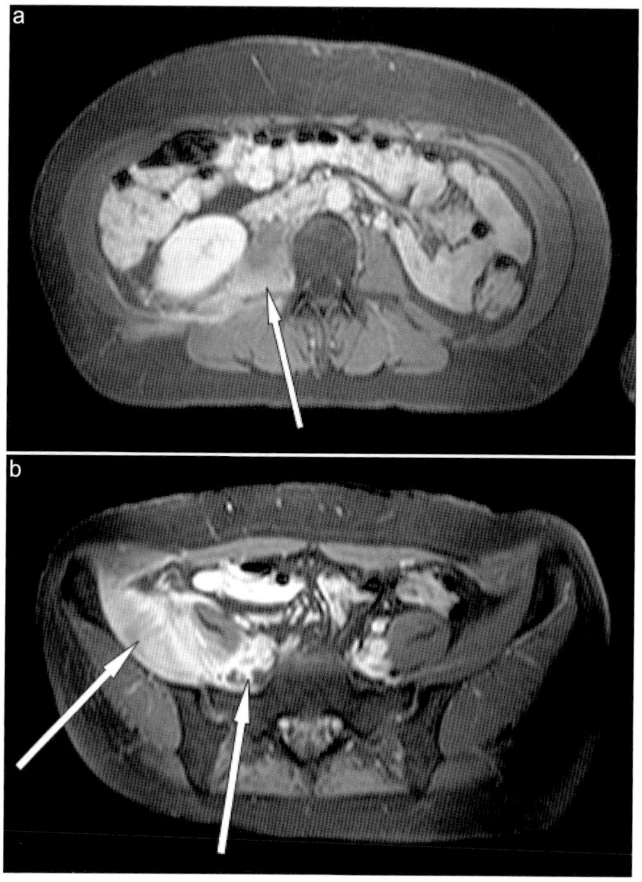

Fig. 1. a, b. MRI of the abdomen. Fibrosis is marked with white arrows.

Retroperitoneal fibrosis is, together with the above-mentioned incidence, a rare disease entity of the retroperitoneal fat where etiology and manifestation are vast. Principally, one divides between primary, idiopathic (Ormond's disease), and secondary retroperitoneal fibrosis.

The secondary type can be caused by radiation, infections, or pharmaceuticals (i.e. Methysegrid). The median age lies between the 5th and 7th decade with a male to female ratio of 3:1. Whereas in the past patients were diagnosed in an advanced state, with symptoms such as azotemia and symmetrical urinary retention, nowadays an early diagnosis can be made by modern imaging methods [4].

In up to 10% of the patients, retroperitoneal fibrosis is associated with an aortic aneurysm, and in 4–8% with a paraneoplastic syndrome. It is crucial to be aware of those coherences

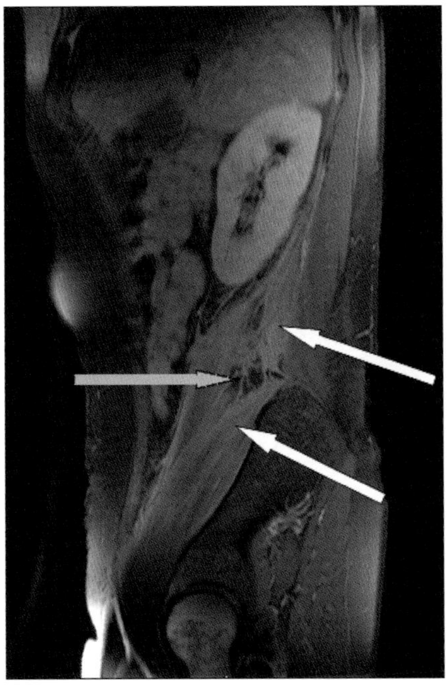

Fig. 2. MRI scan: Normal muscle tissue is marked with a grey arrow. Fibrosis is marked with white arrows.

since an antibiotic therapy should only be started once the diagnostic investigations have been finished [5–7]. Up to 15% of the patients present with a process extending the borders of the retroperitoneum, which complicates diagnosing Ormond's disease; hence, a primary tumor must be considered as one of the differential diagnoses [8].

Our patient presented with right flank pain, which is described as the leading symptom in up to 40% of the cases in the available literature. In addition, back pain, polyuria, nausea, and weight loss are common symptoms [9].

In the CT, the fibrosis is often shown as plaque with the same density as the muscle rather than a diffuse swelling as described in our case. Furthermore, the performed MRI did not show the typical features of a retroperitoneal fibrosis which is distributed along the aorta, vena cava inferior, and both ureters [10, 11]. On the contrary, the MRI described an area of intensification dorsal to the kidney without involving the ureters. Due to this we decided to pursue an open small retroperitoneoscopical approach without relevant risks to obtain a macroscopic impression of the area. It can be discussed if a CT-guided puncture might be a better solution for getting a histological probe.

The results of the clinical examination and of the imaging methods did not show a clear indication for the presence of a retroperitoneal fibrosis. Therefore, we concluded that the surgical exploration was the definitive means in diagnosing retroperitoneal fibrosis by its histopathological and macroscopical results.

Differential diagnosis such as a neoplastic disease should be considered, although lymphomas do not usually present periurethrally. Amyloidosis should also be considered as a differential diagnosis. Imaging can be applied for evaluating differential diagnosis; however, differentiating between malignant and benign entities needs to be assessed by a pathologist. A percutaneous puncture can be an alternative to surgery. We refrained from this method as the surgical exploration benefits from additional information in regard to the macroscopic picture.

Although there are no current guidelines for treating idiopathic retroperitoneal fibrosis, we used an empirically tested pharmaceutical immunosuppression therapy. Corticosteroids and/or tamoxifen are the most commonly used agents, followed by methotrexate [12, 13]. Urological monitoring is vital in the follow-up as the fibrosis can be progressive, leading to required surgery with ureterolysis and intraperitonealization of both ureters. In this context, the above-mentioned association with malignant transformation as a paraneoplastic syndrome should be recognized. The finding of a retroperitoneal fibrosis should not exclude the possibility of an underlying malignant disease. A gastroscopy, colonoscopy, abdominal ultrasound, CT of the abdomen and pelvis, chest x-ray as well as a urological and gynecological consultation should be performed to complete a full investigation, as done in our case study.

Conclusion

On the whole, our case study shows that the surgical exploration and the subsequent histopathological assessment are crucial for diagnosing idiopathic retroperitoneal fibrosis, especially in cases in which non-invasive investigations do not show distinct findings. Nowadays, surgical exploration can be performed via minimally invasive approaches, thereby reducing the surgical trauma to a minimum. The importance of diagnosis and knowledge of the disease, especially its association with malignancy, is crucial in order to offer the right treatment option.

This case study demonstrates that the surgical exploration, the intraoperative macroscopic picture, and the histopathological assessment were the key for diagnosing idiopathic retroperitoneal fibrosis. This led to the successful treatment with immunosuppressive agents, resulting in an arrest of disease progression by 80–90% [12, 13].

Disclosure Statement

Achim Troja, Nader El-Sourani, Dalibur Antolovic and Hans-Rudolph Raab have no conflict of interest.

References

1 Albarran JJ: Rétention rénale par périurérite: libération externe de l'uretère. Ass Fr Urol 1905;9: 511–515.

2 Ormond JK: Bilateral ureteral obstruction due to envelopment and compression by inflammatory retroperitoneal process. J Urol 1948;59:1072–1079.

3 Ormond JK: Idiopathic retroperitoneal fibrosis, an established clinical entity. JAMA 1960;174:1561–1568.

4 Heidenreich A, Derakhshani P, Neubauer S, Krug B: Behandlungsergebnisse der primären und sekundären retroperitonealen Fibrose. Urologe 2000; 39:141–148.

5 Koep L, Zuidema GD: The clinical significance of retroperitoneal fibrosis. Surg 1977;81:250–257.

6 Lepor H, Walsh PC: Idiopathic retroperitoneal fibrosis. J Urol 1979;122:1–6.

7 Parums DV, Choudhury RP, Shields SA, Davies AH: Characterisation of inflammatory cells associated with idiopathic retroperitoneal fibrosis. Br J Urol 1991;67:564–568.

8 Amis ES: Retroperitoneal fibrosis. AJR Am J Roentgenol 1982;157:45–48.

9 Baker LRI, Mallinson WJW, Gregory MC, et al.: Idiopathic retroperitoneal fibrosis. A retrospective analysis of 60 cases. Br J Urol 1988;60:497–503.

10 Bachmann G, Bauer T, Rau WS: MRT und CT in Diagnose und Verlaufskontrolle der idiopathischen retroperitonealen Fibrose. Radiologie 1955; 35:200–207.

11 Kottra JJ, Dunnick NR: Retroperitoneal fibrosis. Radiol Clin North Am 1996;34:1259–1275.

12 Kermani T, Crowson CS, Achenbach SJ, Luthra HS: Idiopathic retroperitoneal fibrosis: a retrospective review of clinical presentation, treatment, and outcomes. Mayo Clin Proc 2011;86:297–303.

13 Swartz RD: Idiopathic retroperitoneal fibrosis: a review of the pathogenesis and approaches to treatment. Am J Kidney Dis 2009;54:546–553.

Viszeralmedizin
Gastrointestinal Medicine and Surgery

Original Article · Originalarbeit

Viszeralmedizin 2013;29:125–130
DOI: 10.1159/000350538

Online publiziert: 12. April 2013

Use of Age-Albumin Ratio as a Single Predictor of 30-Day Mortality after Colectomy

Chih-Chien Chin[a,b] Ching-Ho Yen[c] Wen-Li Hsu[d] Jeng-Yi Wang[a,b] Chia-Hao Chang[e,f]

[a] Section of Colon and Rectal Surgery, Department of Surgery, Chang Gung Memorial Hospital, Chiayi,
[b] Graduate Institute of Clinical Medical Science, College of Medicine, Chang Gung University, Taoyuan,
[c] Department of Industrial Engineering and Management Information, Huafan University, Taipei,
[d] Division of Hematology and Oncology, Department of Medicine, Chang Gung Memorial Hospital,
[e] Department of Nursing,
[f] Chronic Diseases and Health Promotion Research Center, Chang Gung University of Science and Technology, Chiayi, Taiwan

Keywords
Colorectal cancer · Postoperative mortality · Age-albumin ratio · Receiver operating characteristic curve

Summary
Background: Colorectal cancer is among the three leading cancers and causes of mortality worldwide. It is important to develop an effective single-parameter screening technique for reducing the postoperative mortality rate. Previous studies have proved that patient age is a major factor influencing postoperative mortality. A strong association has been reported between serum albumin and patient age. We aimed to identify new predictors on the basis of age-albumin ratio (AAR) for assessing 30-day mortality after colectomy. **Patients and Methods:** Detailed information about patients with colon cancer was retrieved from the Colorectal Section Tumor Registry at Chang Gung Memorial Hospital, Taiwan. The study subjects comprised 3,732 consecutive patients with colon cancer who had undergone elective, potentially curative surgery. **Results:** The area under the receiver operating characteristic curve (AUC) of the AAR was significantly larger than the AUC of serum albumin. The low specificity of AAR was compensated by its substantially high sensitivity. An AAR of ≥20 years g^{-1} nl^{-1} was found to be the most prevalent threshold value. **Conclusion:** The present investigation suggests that AAR can be used in clinical practice as a simple parameter for the identification of patients at risk of 30-day mortality after colectomy.

Schlüsselwörter
Kolorektales Karzinom · Postoperative Mortalität · Alters-Albumin-Ratio · «Receiver Operating Characteristic»-Kurve

Zusammenfassung
Hintergrund: Das kolorektale Karzinom gehört zu den drei führenden Krebserkrankungen und Todesursachen weltweit. Die Entwicklung einer effektiven Ein-Parameter-Screening-Technik zur Reduktion der postoperativen Mortalitätsrate ist bedeutend. Frühere Studien haben belegt, dass das Patientenalter ein wichtiger Faktor für die postoperative Mortalität ist. Ein ausgeprägter Zusammenhang von Serumalbumin und Patientenalter ist festgestellt worden. Wir beabsichtigten daher, auf der Grundlage der Alters-Albumin-Ratio neue Prädiktoren zur Beurteilung der 30-Tage-Mortalität nach Kolektomie zu identifizieren. **Patienten und Methoden:** Detaillierte Informationen zu Patienten mit Dickdarmkrebs wurden aus der Colorectal Section Tumor Registry am Chang Gung Memorial Hospital, Taiwan, abgerufen. Die Probandengruppe setzte sich aus 3732 konsekutiven Patienten mit Dickdarmkrebs zusammen, die sich einer elektiven, potenziell kurativen Operation unterzogen hatten. **Ergebnisse:** Die Fläche unter der «Receiver Operating Characteristic»(ROC)-Kurve der Alters-Albumin-Ratio war signifikant größer als die ROC-Kurve des Serumalbumins. Die geringe Spezifität der Alters-Albumin-Ratio wurde durch deren erheblich höhere Sensitivität ausgeglichen. Eine Alters-Albumin-Ratio ≥20 Jahre g^{-1} nl^{-1} wurde als der am weitesten verbreitete Schwellenwert identifiziert. **Schlussfolgerung:** Die vorliegende Untersuchung deutet darauf hin, dass die Alters-Albumin-Ratio in der klinischen Praxis als einfacher Parameter zur Identifizierung von Patienten mit dem Risiko einer 30-Tage-Mortalität nach Kolektomie verwendet werden kann.

KARGER
Fax +49 761 4 52 07 14
Information@Karger.com
www.karger.com

1662-6664/13/0292-0125$38.00/0

Accessible online at:
www.karger.com/vim

Chia-Hao Chang, Ph.D.
Department of Nursing and Chronic Diseases and Health Promotion Research Center
Chang Gung University of Science and Technology
2, Chia-pu Rd, West Sec. Pu-tz, Chiayi, 613, Taiwan
howellchang@gmail.com

Background

Colorectal cancer is among the three leading cancers and causes of mortality worldwide, with about 1 million new cases and 528,978 deaths reported in 2002 [1–6]. The statistics and publications of the Department of Health of Taiwan indicate that colorectal cancer is the most commonly diagnosed cancer and the third leading cause of cancer-related deaths among both men and women in Taiwan [7]. It is therefore important to plan health care and to identify the risk factors for postoperative mortality in patients with colorectal cancer.

Despite improvements in surgical techniques, a mortality rate of 5–6.5% has been reported for elective colorectal surgery with resection [8–11]. There is strong evidence that malnutrition increases adverse surgical outcome after major elective surgery [12]. Studies have indicated several malnutrition-related risk factors for postoperative mortality [13, 14]. It is well established that hypoalbuminemia (serum albumin level ≤3.5 g/dl), as a marker of malnutrition, is strongly related to a high risk of adverse surgical outcomes [15–18]. Compared with other preoperative parameters, the serum albumin level is a frequently used predictor of malnutrition as well as risk of poor postoperative outcomes in clinical practice. One of the main advantages is the relatively low cost of the serum albumin test [19].

As noted in previous studies, the age of patients with colorectal cancer is another major predictor of adverse surgical outcomes. For example, in a previous study, the patients were divided into age groups of 0–59 years, 60–69 years, 70–79 years, 80 years, and >80 years, and the operative risk significantly increased in the older-age group [20]. Other studies, in which the patients were also divided into several age groups, used odds ratios of postoperative mortality for the different strata of patients. An increasing risk of postoperative mortality is observed with increasing age [21, 22]. Many recent studies can be referred to regarding the association of mortality and age [23–26]. All these studies aimed to discover that an increase in postoperative mortality rates is associated with aging. Overall, preoperative serum albumin level and age can prominently affect the postoperative outcomes of patients with colorectal cancer undergoing surgical treatment [27].

Many studies support the assumption that serum albumin levels decrease with age [28, 29]. The ratio of age to serum albumin can be considered as a single and easy-to-determine index for predicting 30-day mortality; the significance of age can be weighed by dividing it by serum albumin. Use of receiver operating characteristic (ROC) curves is suggested for evaluating the diagnostic value of indices on the basis of a single cut-off value of a continuous variable [30]. Thus, it would be interesting to evaluate whether the application of a new index, based on the ratio of age and serum albumin, will increase the area under the ROC curves (AUC) for assessing 30-day mortality, compared with that of the index based on serum albumin alone. We expected this new index to be more significantly related to 30-day mortality than serum albumin alone. Finally, we attempted to determine the optimal cut-off value of the new index for predicting the risk of 30-day mortality after colectomy.

Table 1. Pathological and clinical characteristics of patients and 30-day mortality

Parameter	Median (IQR)
Age, years	65 (54–74)
Height, cm	159 (153–165)
Weight, kg	59 (52–67)
Preoperative CEA level, ng/ml	3.3 (1.9–7.8)
Serum albumin level, g/nl	4.0 (3.6–4.3)
Hemoglobin level, g%	11.7 (9.8–13.3)
	n = 3,732 (%)
Medical illness – asthma	
Yes	119 (3.19)
No	3,613 (96.81)
Medical illness – diabetes	
Yes	506 (13.56)
No	3,226 (86.44)
Medical illness – liver cirrhosis	
Yes	48 (1.29)
No	3,684 (98.71)
Tumor location	
Right colon	1,449 (38.83)
Left colon	2,283 (61.17)
TNM stage	
I	488 (13.08)
II	1,731 (46.38)
III	1,513 (40.54)
30-day mortality	
Yes	40 (1.07)
No	3,692 (98.93)

IQR = Interquartile range; CEA = carcinoembryonic antigen; TNM = tumor node metastasis.

Methods

Patients

Detailed information about patients with colon cancer, such as patient- and tumor-related factors and follow-up status, was retrieved from the Colorectal Section Tumor Registry (CRSTR) at Chang Gung Memorial Hospital, Taiwan. All the data in this registry were prospectively collected. Patient demographic data, comorbidities, tumor characteristics, and postoperative mortality were included in the data collection. Patient-related factors comprised age, height, weight, hemoglobin level, serum albumin level, carcinoembryonic antigen (CEA) level, and comorbidities. The following comorbidities that may influence the postoperative outcome were recorded in this study: asthma, diabetes, and liver cirrhosis. Tumor-related factors comprised location and stage. Tumors were staged according to the sixth edition of the American Joint Committee on Cancer (AJCC) tumor node metastasis (TNM) staging system. With regard to location, the tumors were categorized as those present in the right colon (from the cecum to the transverse colon) and as those present in the left colon (from the splenic flexure to the sigmoid colon).

The study subjects comprised 3,732 consecutive patients with colon cancer who had undergone elective, potentially curative surgery at the Chang Gung Memorial Hospital from January 1995 to December 2008. Patients with metastatic disease (stage IV colon cancer) were excluded from the study since the treatments for these patients vary and are always palliative. Every patient in this study underwent standard oncological resection of the colon and received routine postoperative care.

Statistical Analyses

The pathological and clinical characteristics of the patients are shown in table 1. To exclude the confounding factors, a logistic regression analysis was performed using a multivariate stepwise selection procedure to analyze the factors that significantly differed between patients with 30-day mortality and non-30-day mortality in the univariate analysis (inclusion factors were those with a p value of <0.05 determined by univariate analysis). The univariate analysis included the Wilcoxon test for medians and chi-square test or Fisher's exact test (if one of the cell counts was small or zero) for discrete data. Moreover, we have discussed the way of feature extraction from the significant factors derived from the logistic regression model (the ratio of the first and second significant factors). In order to determine the way having the strongest association with 30-day mortality, we derived the AUCs for the prediction of 30-day mortality by using each of the candidate predictors. Furthermore, we graphically compared the AUCs and tested the equality of the ROC curves by area test [31]. The main aim was to identify the best predictor of 30-day mortality in terms of sensitivity and specificity. The optimal threshold value (cut-off value) of each candidate predictor was calculated as follows:

$$\text{Optimal cut-off value} = \min\left(\sqrt{(1 - \textit{sensitivity})^2 + (1 - \textit{specificity})^2}\right) \quad (1)$$

Table 2. Surgery-related complications in 40 patients with 30-day mortality

Complications	Incidence
Lung (atelectasis, pneumonia)	15
CV (MI, CVA, embolism)	5
Bladder dysfunction	1
GI (obstruction, bleeding)	4
Anastomosis (leakage, stenosis)	5
Others	6
Combination	4

CV = Cardiovascular; MI = myocardial infarction; CVA = cerebrovascular accident; GI = gastrointestinal.

We determined the sensitivity and specificity for the prediction of 30-day mortality on the basis of the threshold values of the candidate predictors. All the statistical analyses were conducted using the 'MASS' and 'ucR' packages of R 2.9.2 statistical software (R Foundation for Statistical Computing, Vienna, Austria) and Statistical Analysis System (SAS) 9.1.3 software (SAS Institute, Cary, NC, USA).

Results

Demographic Data

The pathological and clinical characteristics of the patients are shown in table 1. The number of patients with 30-day mortality was 40. The morbidity rate was 10.7% in the non-30-day mortality group and 100% in the 30-day mortality group. Surgery-related complications in 40 patients with 30-day mortality are shown in table 2.

Univariate and Multivariate Analyses of 30-Day Mortality

By performing univariate analysis, we found that weight, age, preoperative CEA level, hemoglobin level, serum albumin level, asthma, diabetes, and liver cirrhosis were statistically significant (table 3). With regard to multivariate analysis, age, serum albumin level, and diabetes were found to be the significant predictors. Moreover, the logistic regression model from SAS revealed that patients whose age increased by 10 years, with the other factors remaining constant, were at a 1.852 times higher risk of mortality than the others. Patients whose serum albumin levels increased by one unit (0.1 g/dl), with the other factors remaining constant, were 0.248 (0.146–0.423) times more susceptible to mortality than the others. Similarly, patients with diabetes were 2.668 (1.286–5.542) times more susceptible to mortality than those without diabetes (table 3).

AUCs of Serum Albumin and AAR for the Prediction of 30-Day Mortality

The ratio of the first and second significant factors was age-albumin ratio (AAR) [32]. In order to assess which predictor

Table 3. Comparison of the pathological and clinical characteristics of patients with non-30-day and 30-day mortality

	Univariate analysis		Multivariate analysis		
	Z/odds ratio	p value	odds ratio	95% CI	p value
Height	–1.70	0.089	–	–	–
Weight	–4.09	<0.001	1.000	(0.998–1.003)	0.780
Age	5.66	<0.001	1.064	(1.026–1.103)	0.001
Preoperative CEA level	4.84	<0.001	1.000	(0.996–1.004)	0.947
Hemoglobin level	–2.58	0.010	1.008	(0.928–1.095)	0.853
Serum albumin level	–6.10	<0.001	0.248	(0.146–0.423)	<0.001
Medical illness – asthma	3.46	0.037	2.947	(0.935–9.285)	0.065
Medical illness – diabetes	3.12	0.002	2.668	(1.286–5.542)	0.008
Medical illness – liver cirrhosis	9.21	0.002	3.244	(0.769–13.679)	0.109
Tumor location	0.77	0.420	–	–	–
TNM stage	2.35	0.310	–	–	–

CI = Confidence interval; CEA = carcinoembryonic antigen; TNM = tumor node metastasis.

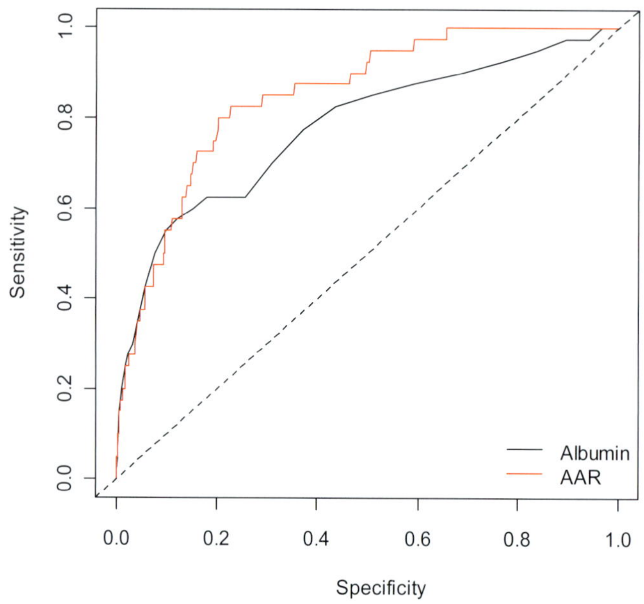

Fig. 1. ROC curves for serum albumin and AAR for the prediction of 30-day mortality.

Table 4. AUCs for the prediction of 30-day mortality, derived on the basis of the threshold values of serum albumin and the new indices

	AUC	p value
Age-albumin ratio	0.851	–
Serum albumin	0.779	0.0002

AUC = Area under the receiver operating characteristic curve.

Table 5. Sensitivity and specificity for the prediction of 30-day mortality, determined on the basis of the threshold values of serum albumin and the new indices

	Sensitivity	Specificity
Serum albumin level of ≤3.5 g/nl	0.625	0.81907
Age-albumin ratio of ≥20 years g^{-1} nl^{-1}	0.800	0.79605

(serum albumin or AAR) was more significantly related to 30-day mortality, we conducted the area test (results shown in table 4). Testing of the difference between serum albumin and AAR showed that the ROC curves for serum albumin and AAR were unequal. AAR had larger AUCs, while serum albumin had a significantly smaller AUC. Figure 1 shows the ROC curves for serum albumin and AAR for the prediction of 30-day mortality. We found that the ROC curve for AAR was almost consistently higher than that for serum albumin.

The values of sensitivity and specificity for the prediction of 30-day mortality, determined on the basis of the threshold values of serum albumin and AAR, are shown in table 5. The sensitivities are as follows: serum albumin level of ≤3.5 g/nl and AAR of ≥20 years g^{-1} nl^{-1}. The specificities are as follows: serum albumin level of ≤3.5 g/nl and AAR of ≥20 years g^{-1} nl^{-1}.

Discussion

Our study has several strengths. To begin with, it is the first study that combined age with serum albumin, forming a new index to evaluate the postoperative 30-day mortality in patients with colon cancer. Additionally, by using AUCs, we were able to examine each (or any) combination of the risk factors to determine the one that was most strongly associated with adverse operative outcomes.

Bad food intake habits contribute to hypoalbuminemia [33]. Food intake was measured by a food frequency questionnaire in our study. Frequency of consumption in the recent 5 years was recorded for the following 12 food items: rice, bread, instant noodles, fish/shrimp, red meat, white meat, viscera, eggs, vegetables, milk, coffee, and fruit. However, we found that all of the 12 items were not statistically significant in regard to mortality. Traditionally, hypoalbuminemia is associated with a high risk of adverse surgical outcomes [15–18]. Serum albumin is a better prognostic predictor of operative outcome than anthropomorphic markers of nutritional status. Older patients often have many coexisting diseases and develop hypoalbuminemia; i.e., serum albumin levels decrease with age, and this association is independent of sex. On the basis of these findings, many studies have suggested preoperative low serum albumin levels and old age as the fundamental factors that increase 30-day mortality after colorectal surgery [8, 24, 25]. In clinical practice, the most important advantage is that the serum albumin test is a relatively low-cost test, and age determination is easy. The AAR is an index that assessed older patients by the stricter criteria. Our results show that the percentage of the AAR of ≥0.8 years g^{-1} nl^{-1} in cases of mortality has higher values (80%). Hence, a combination of the two parameters of age and serum albumin should be used more frequently as a prognostic tool to predict postoperative mortality. Concomitant medical illnesses such as asthma, diabetes, and liver cirrhosis have also been reported in several studies as significant predictors of 30-day mortality [13, 34, 35]. The results of this study are in accordance with those of the studies cited above. Specific postoperative complications were identical in the 30-day mortality group and the non-30-day mortality group. However, there were more pulmonary complications in the 30-day mortality group than in the non-30-day mortality group (37.5 vs. 0.4%; $p < 0.001$). This implies that postoperative pulmonary complications are frequent in terms of 30-day mortality. Moreover, serum albumin level and the patient's age were parameters having a high correlation with pulmonary complications [23, 36]. In our study, means of AAR were compared in both groups. The values were significantly different between those with and without pulmonary complication (16.54 ± 5.16 vs. 26.65 ± 7.81; $p < 0.001$). In multivariate analysis, among the patient-related factors and co-

Table 6. Percentage of the considered measurements in cases of morbidity and mortality

	Percentage, %					
	lung	CV	bladder dysfunction	GI	anastomosis	mortality
Albumin of ≤3.5 g/nl	75.9	42.9	45.8	18.2	31.3	62.5
AAR of ≥20 years g^{-1} nl^{-1}	86.2	42.9	50.8	23.6	29.2	80.0

AAR = Age-albumin ratio; CV = cardiovascular; GI = gastrointestinal.

morbidities, preoperative serum albumin level, age, and diabetes were observed to be markedly associated with the postoperative 30-day mortality in patients with colon cancer. Furthermore, patients whose serum albumin levels increased by one unit (0.1 g/dl), with the other factors remaining constant, were 0.248 times more susceptible to mortality than the others. The risk of 30-day mortality was 1.852 times higher in patients whose age increased by 10 years than in others. Similarly, patients with diabetes were 2.668 times more susceptible to mortality than those without diabetes.

The present study mainly showed that combining two continuous predictors (preoperative serum albumin level and age) significantly affected the prediction of postoperative mortality in patients with colon cancer. In this study, we proposed the use of AAR as a screening parameter for identifying the optimal cut-off value in order to predict the 30-day mortality after colon surgery. AAR of ≥20 years g^{-1} nl^{-1} yielded the minimal value of

$$\sqrt{(1-\mathit{sensitivity})^2+(1-\mathit{specificity})^2} \tag{2}$$

for predicting 30-day mortality. The low specificity was compensated by its substantially high sensitivity. In other words, the new index would offer built-in solutions for situations in which individuals with high risks of 30-day mortality are falsely assumed to have no risk. Moreover, the optimal cut-off values recommended in this study for AAR showed a balance of sensitivity and specificity for the prediction of 30-day mortality (table 5).

Table 6 shows the percentage of the considered measurements in cases of morbidity and mortality. For 30-day mortality, AAR of ≥0.8 years g^{-1} nl^{-1} has higher values (80%) than serum albumin of ≤3.5 g/nl (62.5%), mGPS (modified Glasgow prognostic score) of ≥1 (52.5%), and mGPS of ≥2 (32.5%). For pulmonary complications, AAR of ≥0.8 years g^{-1} nl^{-1} has a higher value (86.2%) than serum albumin of ≤3.5 g/nl (75.9%), mGPS of ≥1 (65.5%), and mGPS of ≥2 (51.7%). This result implies that the use of a combination of serum albumin and age as the predictor of postoperative 30-day mortality in patients with colon cancer is better than that of serum albumin or mGPS alone.

On the basis of the AUCs derived for the prediction of 30-day mortality in patients with colon cancer, we suggest that AAR is a better predictor than serum albumin in Taiwanese subjects. In conclusion, hypoalbuminemia often reflects malnourishment in patients [37]. In the meta-analysis of Braunschweig et al., malnourished patients benefited from parenteral nutrition in terms of mortality [38, 39]. Such an approach has also been shown to reduce the postoperative complication rate by as much as 10% [40]. Hence, in order to reduce AAR as low as possible, our aim should be to initiate preoperative total parenteral nutrition for malnourished colon cancer patients.

Acknowledgment

This study was supported by a grant provided from the Chang Gung Memorial Hospital Research Program (CMRPF680021).

Disclosure Statement

The authors declare that there are no conflicts of interest.

References

1 Parkin DM: International variation. Oncogene 2004;23:6329–6340.
2 Parkin DM, Bray F, Ferlay J, Pisani P: Global cancer statistics, 2002. CA Cancer J Clin 2005;55:74–108.
3 Stal A, Stembalska A, Śmigiel R, Tarkowski R, Grzebieniak Z, Sąsiadek M: Hereditary nonpolyposis colorectal cancer in Lower Silesia. Pol Przegl Chir 2007;79:182–189.
4 Winawer SJ: Colorectal cancer screening. Best Pract Res Clin Gastroenterol 2007;21:1031–1048.
5 Jemal A, Siegel R, Ward E, Hao Y, Xu J, Murray T, Thun MJ: Cancer statistics. CA Cancer J Clin 2008;58:71–96.
6 Center MM, Jemal A, Smith RA, Ward E: Worldwide variations in colorectal cancer. CA Cancer J Clin 2009;59:366–378.
7 *www.doh.gov.tw/statistic/index.htm.*
8 Longo WE, Virgo KS, Johnson FE, Oprian CA, Vernava AM, Wade TP, Phelan MA, Henderson WG, Daley J, Khuri SF: Risk factors for morbidity and mortality after colectomy for colon cancer. Dis Colon Rectum 2000;43:83–91.
9 Ansari MZ, Collopy BT, Hart WG, Carson NJ, Chandraraj EJ: In-hospital mortality and associated complications after bowel surgery in Victorian public hospitals. Aust N Z J Surg 2000;70:6–10.

10 Sjo OH, Larsen S, Lunde OC, Nesbakken A: Short term outcome after emergency and elective surgery for colon cancer. Colorectal Dis 2008;11:733–739.
11 Frederiksen BL, Osler M, Harling H, Danish Colorectal Cancer Group, Ladelund S, Jørgensen T: The impact of socioeconomic factors on 30-day mortality following elective colorectal cancer surgery: a nationwide study. Eur J Cancer 2009;45: 1248–1256.
12 Lohsiriwat V, Chinswangwatanakul V, Lohsiriwat S, Akaraviputh T, Boonnuch W, Methasade A, Lohsiriwat D: Hypoalbuminemia is a predictor of delayed postoperative bowel function and poor surgical outcomes in right-sided colon cancer patients. Asia Pac J Clin Nutr 2007;16:213–217.
13 Mullen JL, Buzby GP, Waldman MT, Gertner MH, Hobbs CL, Rosato EF: Prediction of operative morbidity and mortality by preoperative nutritional assessment. Surg Forum 1979;30:80–82.
14 Ondrula DP, Nelson RL, Prasad ML, Coyle BW, Abcarian H: Multifactorial index of preoperative risk factors in colon resections. Dis Colon Rectum 1992;35:117–122.
15 Bauer J, Capra S: Comparison of a malnutrition screening tool with subjective global assessment in hospitalised patients with cancer – sensitivity and specificity. Asia Pac J Clin Nutr 2003;12:257–260.
16 Sungurtekin H, Sungurtekin U, Balci C, Zencir M, Erdem E: The influence of nutritional status on complications after major intraabdominal surgery. J Am Coll Nutr 2004;23:227–232.
17 Miner TJ, Brennan MF, Jaques DP: A prospective, symptom related, outcomes analysis of 1022 palliative procedures for advanced cancer. Ann Surg 2004;240:719–726.
18 Inoue Y, Miki C, Kusunoki M: Nutritional status and cytokine-related protein breakdown in elderly patients with gastrointestinal malignancies. J Surg Oncol 2004;86:91–98.
19 Gibbs J, Cull W, Henderson W, Daley J, Hur K, Khuri SF: Preoperative serum albumin level as a predictor of operative mortality and morbidity: results from the National VA Surgical Risk Study. Arch Surg 1999;134:36–42.
20 Damhuis RA, Tilanus HW: The influence of age on resection rates and postoperative mortality in 2773 patients with gastric cancer. Eur J Cancer 1995; 31A:928–931.
21 Yancik R, Wesley MN, Ries LAG, Havlik RJ, Long S, Edwards BK, Yates JW: Comorbidity and age as predictors of risk for early mortality of male and female colon carcinoma patients: a population-based study. Cancer 1998;82:2123–2134.
22 Heriot AG, Tekkis PP, Smith JJ, Cohen CRG, Montgomery A, Audisio RA, Thompson MR, Stamatakis JD: Prediction of postoperative mortality in elderly patients with colorectal cancer. Dis Colon Rectum 2006;49:816–824.
23 Marusch F, Koch A, Schmidt U, Steinert R, Ueberrueck T, Bittner R, Berg E, Engemann R, Gellert K, Arbogast R, Körner T, Köckerling F, Gastinger I, Lippert H; Working Group Colon/Rectum Cancer: The impact of the risk factor 'age' on the early postoperative results of surgery for colorectal carcinoma and its significance for perioperative management. World J Surg 2005;29:1013–1021.
24 Alves A, Panis Y, Mathieu P, Mantion G, Kwiatkowski F, Slim K; Association Française de Chirurgie: Postoperative mortality and morbidity in French patients undergoing colorectal surgery: results of a prospective multicenter study. Arch Surg 2005;140:278–283.
25 Alves A, Panis Y, Mantion G, Slim K, Kwiatkowski F, Vicaut E: The AFC score: validation of a 4-item predicting score of postoperative mortality after colorectal resection for cancer or diverticulitis. Results of a prospective multicenter study in 1049 patients. Ann Surg 2007;246:91–96.
26 Gurevitch AJ, Davidovitch B, Kashtan H: Outcome of right colectomy for cancer in octogenarians. J Gastrointest Surg 2009;13:100–104.
27 Sun LC, Chu KS, Cheng SC, Lu CY, Kuo CH, Hsieh JS, Shih YL, Chang SJ, Wang JY: Preoperative serum carcinoembryonic antigen, albumin and age are supplementary to UICC staging systems in predicting survival for colorectal cancer patients undergoing surgical treatment. BMC Cancer 2009; 9:288.
28 Klonoff-Cohen H, Barrett-Connor EL, Edelstein SL: Albumin levels as a predictor of mortality in the healthy elderly. J Clin Epidemiol 1992;45: 207–212.
29 Baumgartner RN, Koehler KM, Romero L, Garry PJ: Serum albumin is associated with skeletal muscle in elderly men and women. Am J Clin Nutr 1996;64:552–558.
30 Kestler HA: ROC with confidence – a Perl program for receiver operator characteristic curves. Comput Methods Programs Biomed 2001;64:133–136.
31 DeLong ER, DeLong DM, Clarke-Pearson DL: Comparing the areas under two or more correlated receiver operating characteristic curves: a nonparametric approach. Biometrics 1988;44:837–845.
32 Chang CH, Yen CH, Chen MY: Using principal component analysis to develop a single-parameter screening tool for metabolic syndrome. BMC Public Health 2010;10:708–715.
33 Norman K, Lochs H, Pirlich M: Malnutrition as a prognostic factor. Chir Gastroenterol 2004;20: 175–180.
34 Agarwal N, Acevedo F, Leighton LS, Cayten CG, Pitchumoni CS: Predictive ability of various nutritional variables for mortality in elderly people. Am J Clin Nutr 1988;48:1173–1178.
35 Apelgren KN, Rombeau JL, Twomey PL, Miller RA: Comparison of nutritional indices and outcome in critically ill patients. Crit Care Med 1982; 10:305–307.
36 Fan ST, Lau WY, Yip WC, Poon GP, Yeung C, Lam WK, Wong KK: Prediction of postoperative pulmonary complications in oesophagogastric surgery. Br J Surg 1987;74:408–410.
37 Fuhrman MP, Charney P, Mueller CM: Hepatic proteins and nutrition assessment. J Am Diet Assoc 2004;104:1258–1264.
38 Braunschweig CL, Levy P, Sheean PM, Wang X: Enteral compared with parenteral nutrition: a meta-analysis. Am J Clin Nutr 2001;74:534–542.
39 Hsu SD, Yu JC, Chen TW, Chou SJ, Hsieh HF, Chan DC: Role of nasogastric tube insertion after gastrectomy. Chir Gastroenterol 2007;23:303–306.
40 Torosian MH: Perioperative nutrition support for patients undergoing gastrointestinal surgery: critical analysis and recommendations. World J Surg 1999;23:565–569.

Viszeralmedizin 29| 2 | 13

Takeda beantragt Genehmigung für das Inverkehrbringen von Vedolizumab gegen mäßig bis stark aktive Colitis ulcerosa und Morbus Crohn in der Europäischen Union

Takeda Pharmaceutical Company Limited («Takeda») gab Anfang März 2013 bekannt, dass das Unternehmen bei der Europäischen Arzneimittel-Agentur (EMA) einen Zulassungsantrag (MAA, Marketing Authorization Application) für Vedolizumab eingereicht hat, einem experimentellen, darmspezifischen, humanisierten, monoklonalen Antikörper zur Behandlung von Erwachsenen mit mäßig bis stark aktiver Colitis ulcerosa (UC) und Morbus Crohn (MC), den beiden häufigsten Formen chronisch-entzündlicher Darmerkrankungen (CED). Nach Zulassung wäre Vedolizumab das erste und einzige darmspezifische Biologikum gegen UC und MC auf dem Markt.

«Colitis ulcerosa und Morbus Crohn sind chronische, kräftezehrende Erkrankungen, gegen die es so gut wie keine wirksame Therapie gibt. Betroffen sind häufig junge Menschen in ihren besten Jahren», sagte Asit Parikh, M.D., Ph.D., Vice President General Medicine bei Takeda (Abb. 1). «Die Ergebnisse von GEMINI, einer Phase-III-Studie zu Vedolizumab, sind vielversprechend. An dieser klinischen Studie nahmen rund 3000 Patienten in nahezu 40 Ländern teil. Damit ist sie die bis heute umfangreichste klinische Studie zu CED.»

Weltweit leiden fast vier Millionen Menschen an CED, davon in der EU mehr als 500 000 an UC und ca. 230 000 an MC. UC und MC sind chronische Erkrankungen, die Entzündungen an den Schleimhäuten des Verdauungstrakts hervorrufen. Von Entzündungen bei MC können verschiedene Areale des Verdauungstrakts betroffen sein, UC befällt ausschließlich den Dickdarm. MC und UC können schmerzhaft und kräftezehrend sein; dies führt unter Umständen zu schwerwiegenden Komplikationen und zu beträchtlichen Einschränkungen der Lebensqualität der Patienten.

Der Zulassungsantrag stützt sich auf die Phase-III-Studien GEMINI I, GEMINI II, GEMINI III und GEMINI LTS (Long-Term Safety/langfristige Sicherheit); diese sind Teil der GEMINI Studies(TM), einem aus vier Studien bestehenden klinischen Programm zur Untersuchung der Wirksamkeit und Sicherheit von Vedolizumab gemessen an klinischem Ansprechen und Remission bei Patienten mit mäßig bis stark aktiver UC und MC, bei denen zumindest eine herkömmliche oder Anti-TNF-alpha-Therapie erfolglos war.

«Durch den spezifischen Wirkungsmechanismus ist Vedolizumab klinisch vielversprechend als Therapiemöglichkeit für Patienten mit mäßig bis stark aktiver UC und MC», sagte Professor Paul Rutgeerts von der katholischen Universität Löwen, Belgien. «Es ist keine Therapie bekannt, die diese Erkrankungen heilen kann; es besteht Bedarf an neuen Behandlungsoptionen für MC und UC, damit Patienten weitere Therapien erhalten, die die Symptome abschwächen und Remissionen ermöglichen.»

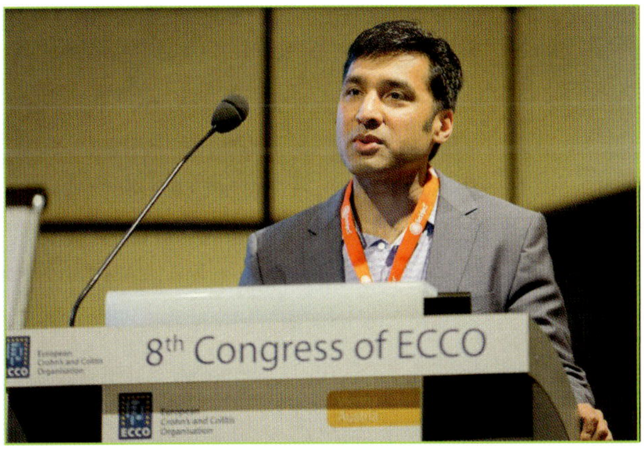

Abb. 1. «UC und MC sind chronische Erkrankungen, gegen die es so gut wie keine wirksame Therapie gibt. Die Studienergebnisse zu Vedolizumab sind vielversprechend», erläutert Vice President General Medicine M.D., Ph.D. Asit Parikh.

Weitere Informationen bei
Ketchum Pleon GmbH
Nicole Kromayer
Theresienhöhe 12, 80339 München
Tel. +49 89 59042-1207, Fax -238
Nicole.Kromayer@ketchumpleon.com

Ticker+++ Ticker+++ Ticker+++ Ticker+++ Ticker+++ Ticker+++ Ticker+++

Bayer. Beim diesjährigen ASCO-GI-Kongress wurden neue Daten zum Krebsmedikament Regorafenib vorgestellt. Darunter sind neue Analysen aus der zulassungsrelevanten Phase-III-Studie CORRECT mit Regorafenib bei metastasiertem Darmkrebs sowie Ergebnisse einer Phase-I-Studie von Regorafenib bei hepatozellulärem Karzinom. Regorafenib wurde im September 2012 auf Basis der CORRECT-Ergebnisse von der Gesundheitsbehörde FDA (USA) unter dem Handelsnamen Stivarga® zur Behandlung von mCRC zugelassen.

Bayer Pharma AG
Anna Koch
anna.koch@bayer.com

Humedics. Der Spezialist für die akute und mobile Messung der individuellen Leberfunktion am Patientenbett hat eine klinische Phase-III-Studie gestartet. Das Hauptziel der Studie besteht darin, mithilfe des LiMAx-Tests schneller risikoarme Patienten nach einer Teilentfernung der Leber zu identifizieren und dadurch das Patientenmanagement zu verbessern. Nach Initiierung der ersten Studienzentren sind bereits erste Patienten in die Studie aufgenommen worden.

Humedics GmbH
Erwin de Buijzer
info@humedics.de

Ziehm Imaging. Es gibt eine neue Generation mobiler C-Bögen von Ziehm Imaging: Die Ziehm Vision Familie kommt mit optimiertem Design, innovativen Funktionen und SmartDose Dosisreduzierung für den vielseitigen Einsatz bis hin zur minimalinvasiven Gefäßchirurgie. Mit SmartDose sind bei optimaler intraoperativer Bildgebung bereits durch den Einsatz hardwarebasierter Filter und Algorithmen bis zu 20% Dosiseinsparung möglich.

Ziehm Imaging
Martin Herzmann
Martin.Herzmann@ziehm-eu.com

KARGER
Fax + 49 761 4 52 07 14
Information@karger.com
www.karger.com

Palliative mCRC-KRAS-wt-Patienten:

30 Monate medianes Gesamtüberleben dank intensiver Erstlinientherapie mit Cetuximab + FOLFIRI

Bei Patienten mit metastasiertem Kolorektalkarzinom (mCRC) und KRAS-Wildtyp kann eine intensive Erstlinientherapie bestehend aus Standardchemotherapie und dem EGFR-Antikörper Cetuximab Vorteile bringen. Prof. Dirk Arnold, Freiburg, erläuterte auf der DGHO-Jahrestagung im Oktober 2012 den Stellenwert der Therapieoption unter anderem anhand der Erbitux®-Zulassungsstudie CRYSTAL: Insgesamt 1198 therapienaive Patienten erhielten im Verhältnis 1:1 randomisiert entweder eine Behandlung mit einer Standardchemotherapie (FOLFIRI) oder eine Kombination mit Cetuximab. Im Vergleich zur alleinigen Chemotherapie ermöglichte die Zugabe des Antikörpers in der retrospektiven Analyse der 666 KRAS-wt-Patienten eine signifikante Verbesserung im Gesamtansprechen (ORR: 57,3 vs. 39,7 %; p < 0,001) und eine signifikante Verbesserung des medianen Gesamtüberlebens (OS: 23,5 vs. 20,0 Monate; p = 0,0093). Die Tumorreduktion führte zu einer Verringerung der Symptome und bot die Chance auf Resektion.

Eine retrospektive Subgruppenanalyse der CRYSTAL-Studie zeigte außerdem, dass die Kombination FOLFIRI + Cetuximab eine maximale Symptomlinderung nach bereits 8 Wochen zeigte – im Vergleich zu 16 Wochen bei FOLFIRI alleine. Das Erreichen einer frühen Tumorschrumpfung (≥20% innerhalb von 8 Wochen) habe neben dem direkten klinischen Nutzen auch einen hohen prognostischen Stellenwert, so Arnold. Denn im Vergleich zu Patienten ohne frühe Tumorreduktion um ≥20% profitierten Patienten mit früher Tumorschrumpfung von einem im Durchschnitt 11,4 Monate längeren Gesamtüberleben (30,0 vs. 18,6 Monate; p < 0,001). Fast zwei Drittel (62%) der mit der Cetuximab-Kombination behandelten KRAS-wt-Patienten erreichten eine frühe Tumorschrumpfung ≥20%, unter FOLFIRI allein war dies nur bei der Hälfte (49%) der Fall. Der Einsatz des Biomarkers KRAS sowie des klinischen Markers «frühe Tumorschrumpfung» ermöglicht somit eine frühe Prognoseabschätzung.

Literaturangaben und weitere
Informationen bei
Merck Serono GmbH
Yvonne Weißhuhn
Alsfelder Straße 17
64289 Darmstadt
yvonne.weisshuhn@external.merckgroup.com

Adalimumab zur Behandlung des schweren, aktiven pädiatrischen Morbus Crohn zugelassen

Im November 2012 erhielt Adalimumab (Humira®) die Zulassung zur Behandlung des pädiatrischen Morbus Crohn. Der TNF-Inhibitor ist indiziert zur Behandlung von Kindern und Jugendlichen zwischen 6 und 17 Jahren mit schwerem, aktivem Morbus Crohn, die nur unzureichend auf konventionelle Therapien angesprochen haben, die eine Unverträglichkeit gegenüber einer solchen Therapie haben oder bei denen eine solche Therapie kontraindiziert ist. Damit ist Adalimumab der erste selbst-applizierbare TNF-Inhibitor in dieser Indikation.

Basis der Zulassung sind die Daten der 52-wöchigen, multizentrischen, randomisierten, doppelblinden klinischen Phase-III-Studie IMAgINE 1 [1]. Sie untersuchte körpergewichtsbasiert 2 Dosierungen von Adalimumab hinsichtlich der Remissionsinduktion und -erhaltung bei 192 pädiatrischen Patienten mit mittelschwerem bis schwerem, aktivem Morbus Crohn, bei denen die konventionelle Behandlung nicht erfolgreich war. Die Patienten waren zwischen 6 und 17 Jahre alt und wiesen einen Pediatric Crohn's Disease Activity Index (PCDAI) Score > 30 auf. Alle Studienteilnehmer erhielten als Induktionstherapie offen Adalimumab in den Wochen 0 und 2 (160 mg/80 mg bei einem Körpergewicht (KG) ≥ 40 kg bzw. 80 mg/40 mg bei KG < 40 kg). In Woche 4 wurden 188 Patienten nach ihrem Ansprechen und vorheriger Infliximab-Exposition stratifiziert und anschließend randomisiert 2 Adalimumab-Dosierungen zugeteilt. Patienten der Gruppe mit der höheren Adalimumab-Dosis (Standard-Erhaltungsdosis) erhielten über 48 Wochen 40 mg (≥40 kg KG) bzw. 20 mg (<40 kg KG) alle 2 Wochen. In der niedrigdosierten Adalimumab-Gruppe wurden 20 mg bzw. 10 mg (je nach KG ≥ oder <40 kg) 14-tägig subkutan als Erhaltungstherapie verabreicht. Zur Woche 26 erreichten 39% der Patienten mit der Standard-Erhaltungsdosis eine klinische Remission, zur Woche 52 33% der Patienten mit der Standard-Erhaltungsdosis. Die Sicherheitsdaten der Studie entsprachen dem bekannten Sicherheitsprofil aus anderen Indikationen.

Literatur

1 Hyams J et al.: Gastroenterology 2012;143(2):365–374.

Weitere Informationen bei
AbbVie Deutschland GmbH & Co.KG
Maren Nienstedt
Max-Planck-Ring 2a, 65205 Wiesbaden
maren.nienstedt@abbvie.com

Ticker+++ Ticker+++ Ticker+++ Ticker+++ Ticker+++ Ticker+++ Ticker+++

Roche. Wird der Angiogenese-Hemmer Bevacizumab bei Patienten mit metastasiertem kolorektalem Karzinom (mCRC) kontinuierlich in der Erst- und in der Zweitlinientherapie gegeben, jeweils kombiniert mit einer 5-FU-basierten Chemotherapie, so verlängert dies das Gesamtüberleben signifikant. Der Arzt ist künftig in der Lage, seinen Patienten mit mCRC eine weitere Therapielinie mit Bevacizumab anzubieten.

Roche Pharma AG
Ulla Satzger
ulla.satzger@roche.com

Olympus. Beim 15. Internationalen Endoskopie-Symposium in Düsseldorf präsentierten mehr als 30 international renommierte Experten rund 1800 Teilnehmern aus über 50 Ländern die aktuellen Fortschritte in der Endoskopie. Bei der vom Kongresspartner Olympus unterstützten Auftakt-Pressekonferenz stellten Prof. Neuhaus, PD Dr. Schumacher und Prof. Sung die Anwendung neuer Endoskopieverfahren bei Erkrankungen des Verdauungstraktes und die Evaluierung hinsichtlich ihres klinischen Nutzens vor.

John Warning Corporate Communications GmbH
Martina John
m.john@johnwarning.de

Daiichi Sankyo. Der 1. Patient wurde in die weltweite Phase-III-Studie METIV-HCC mit Tivantinib (ARQ 197) eingeschlossen. Tivantinib ist ein in klinischer Prüfung befindlicher selektiver Inhibitor der Rezeptortyrosinkinase c-MET. Die Substanz befindet sich in der letzten Phase der klinischen Entwicklung. Sie wird in der Therapie von Patienten mit hepatozellulärem Karzinom (HCC), die bereits systemisch vorbehandelt sind, untersucht.

Daiichi Sankyo Deutschland GmbH
Pia Nothing
pia.nothing@daiichi-sankyo.de

Fax + 49 761 4 52 07 14
Information@karger.com
www.karger.com

Viszeralmedizin
Gastrointestinal Medicine and Surgery

Tagungen und Kongresse · Meetings and Conferences

Viszeralmedizin 2013;29:134–135

30.04.–03.05.2013 **München** Deutschland	**130. Kongress der Deutschen Gesellschaft für Chirurgie**	**Auskunft:** www.chirurgie2013.de
03.05.–04.05.2013 **Frankfurt/Main** Deutschland	**22. Kongress der Mitteldeutschen Gesellschaft für Gastroenterologie**	**Auskunft:** www.mgfg.de
04.05.2013 **München** Deutschland	**Falk Gastro-Forum: Therapeutische Herausforderungen 2013 in Gastroenterologie und Hepatologie**	**Auskunft:** www.falkfoundation.de
30.05.–01.06.2013 **Wien** Österreich	**54. Österreichischer Chirurgenkongress (ÖGC-Jahrestagung)**	**Auskunft:** www.chirurgenkongress.at
01.06.2013 **Berlin** Deutschland	**Falk Gastro-Forum: Frühe gastrointestinale Tumore**	**Auskunft:** www.falkfoundation.de
06.06.–08.06.2013 **Graz** Österreich	**39. Gemeinsame Tagung der Österreichischen Gesellschaft für Urologie und Andrologie und der Bayerischen Urologenvereinigung**	**Auskunft:** www.uro2013.at
07.06.–08.06.2013 **Hamburg** Deutschland	**Anorektaler Endo-Sonographiekurs – Grund- und Aufbaukurs**	**Auskunft:** www.enddarm-zentrum.de
07.06.2013 **Frankfurt/Main** Deutschland	**Kapsel-Klub: Kurs zur Dünndarm-Kapselendoskopie**	**Auskunft:** www.dgvs.de
07.06.–08.06.2013 **Stuttgart** Deutschland	**Falk Symposium 188: Inflammatory Bowel Diseases: Microbiota versus the Barrier**	**Auskunft:** www.falkfoundation.de
13.06.–15.06.2013 **Lüneburg** Deutschland	**Falk Seminar: VII. Lüneburger Gastroenterologisches Seminar**	**Auskunft:** www.falkfoundation.de
13.06.–15.06.2013 **Baden-Baden** Deutschland	**54. Jahrestagung der Südwestdeutschen Gesellschaft für Urologie**	**Auskunft:** www.swdgu.de/2013
14.06.–15.06.2013 **Köln** Deutschland	**2. Hepatologie-Update-Seminar**	**Auskunft:** www.hepato-update.com
14.06.–15.06.2013 **Hamburg** Deutschland	**SommerGespräche: Der onkologische Patient im Mittelpunkt**	**Auskunft:** www.nationalegesundheitsakademie.de
21.06.–22.06.2013 **Hannover** Deutschland	**10. HepNet Symposium**	**Auskunft:** www.deutsche-leberstiftung.de
22.06.2013 **Frankfurt/Main** Deutschland	**Falk Gastro-Forum: Update Therapiestrategie Darm + Leber**	**Auskunft:** www.falkfoundation.de
24.06.–26.06.2013 **Altötting** Deutschland	**90. Jahrestagung der Vereinigung der Bayerischen Chirurgen e.V.**	**Auskunft:** www.mcn-nuernberg.de

KARGER
Fax +49 761 4 52 07 14
Information@Karger.com
www.karger.com

Accessible online at:
www.karger.com/vim

28.06.–29.06.2013 **Hannover** Deutschland	**3. International Symposium on Complications in GI Endoscopy**	**Auskunft:** www.complications-in-endoscopy.com
29.06.2013 **Wuppertal** Deutschland	**Falk Gastro-Forum: Schnittstellen in der Inneren Medizin – Gastroenterologie/Hepatologie/Onkologie/Kardiologie**	**Auskunft:** www.falkfoundation.de
06.07.2013 **Chemnitz** Deutschland	**Falk Gastro-Forum: Der akut erkrankte gastroenterologische Patient**	**Auskunft:** www.falkfoundation.de
25.08.–29.08.2013 **München** Deutschland	**35th Annual Conference of the International Society for Clinical Biostatistics**	**Auskunft:** www.iscb2013.info
05.09.2013 **Graz** Österreich	**Falk Workshop: GERD – Gastroesophageal Reflux Disease**	**Auskunft:** www.falkfoundation.de
06.09.–07.09.2013 **Graz** Österreich	**Falk Symposium: Eosinophilic Esophagitis: A Novel Chronic-Inflammatory Disease of the GI Tract**	**Auskunft:** www.falkfoundation.de
11.09.–14.09.2013 **Nürnberg** Deutschland	**Viszeralmedizin 2013**	**Auskunft:** www.dgvs.de
21.09.2013 **Ulm** Deutschland	**Falk Gastro-Forum: Gastroenterologie und Hepatologie 2013. Von der Empirie zur «Personalisierten Medizin» – eine Standortbestimmung**	**Auskunft:** www.falkfoundation.de
25.09.–28.09.2013 **Dresden** Deutschland	**65. Kongress der Deutschen Gesellschaft für Urologie e.V**	**Auskunft:** www.dgu-kongress.de
02.10.–03.10.2013 **London** England	**Falk Symposium 190 (Part I): Challenges in the Care of IBD in Patients of All Ages**	**Auskunft:** www.falkfoundation.de
04.10.–05.10.2013 **London** England	**VI Falk Gastro-Conference (Part II): Liver Diseases in 2013: Advances in Pathogenesis and Treatment**	**Auskunft:** www.falkfoundation.de
11.10.–12.10.2013 **Dresden** Deutschland	**ElbeGespräche: Der onkologische Patient im Mittelpunkt**	**Auskunft:** www.nationalegesundheitsakademie.de
13.10.–16.10.2013 **Berlin** Deutschland	**4th World Congress of Pediatric Surgeons: Children's Surgery with Competence & Heart**	**Auskunft:** www.wofaps2013.com
08.11.–09.11.2013 **Tübingen** Deutschland	**WinterGespräche: Der onkologische Patient im Mittelpunkt**	**Auskunft:** www.nationalegesundheitsakademie.de
09.11.2013 **Braunschweig** Deutschland	**Falk Gastro-Forum: Divertikelkrankheit**	**Auskunft:** www.falkfoundation.de
29.11.–30.11.2013 **Augsburg** Deutschland	**endo-update 2013**	**Auskunft:** www.endoupdate.de
06.12.–07.12.2013 **Essen** Deutschland	**5. Deutsches Robotisches Urologie-Symposium**	**Auskunft:** www.dgru.de
19.02.–23.02.2014 **Berlin** Deutschland	**31. Deutscher Krebskongress (DKK)**	**Auskunft:** www.krebsgesellschaft.de
25.03.–28.03.2014 **Berlin** Deutschland	**131. Kongress der Deutschen Gesellschaft für Chirurgie**	**Auskunft:** www.chirurgie2014.de

Viszeralmedizin
Gastrointestinal Medicine and Surgery

Hinweise für Autoren

Viszeralmedizin 2013;29

Einreichung von Manuskripten
Die Zeitschrift «Viszeralmedizin» ist ein Forum für die interdisziplinäre Diskussion aller wichtigen und aktuellen Themen der Viszeralchirurgie, Gastroenterologie und Hepatologie.

Manuskripte sind zu senden an:

S. Karger Verlag für Medizin und Naturwissenschaften GmbH
Alexander Eitner
Postfach
79095 Freiburg (Deutschland)
Tel. +49 761 45 20 730
Fax +49 761 45 20 714
a.eitner@karger.com

Sprache
Die Beiträge können in deutscher oder englischer Sprache (amerikanische oder britische Rechtschreibung) eingereicht werden.

Rubriken und Umfang
Die Manuskripte sollen in 1 1/2-zeiligem Abstand mit beidseitig je 3 cm Rand, Schrift 12 pt eingereicht werden.

Folgender Umfang sollte nicht überschritten werden:

	Druckseiten	Entspricht Zeichen*
Hauptthema	5	30 000
Interdisziplinäres Gespräch	5	30 000
Übersichtsarbeit, Originalarbeit	5	30 000
Kasuistik	5	18 000
Brief an die Herausgeber	2	12 000
Übrige Beiträge	2	12 000

***Einschließlich deutscher und englischer Zusammenfassung, Abbildungen, Tabellen und Literaturzitate. Pro Tabelle und Abbildung werden pauschal 1500 Zeichen gezählt.**

Für Umfangsüberschreitungen wird dem Autor ein Mehrkostenanteil in Rechnung gestellt.

Bedingungen
Über die Annahme wissenschaftlicher Beiträge wird aufgrund mehrerer Gutachten entschieden (peer-review).
Der Verlag geht davon aus, dass eingereichte Manuskripte weder gleichzeitig bei einem anderen Journal begutachtet werden noch bereits ganz oder teilweise anderswo publiziert sind. Die Einreichung eines Beitrags impliziert, dass die Autoren alleinige Inhaber des Copyrights sind und dass der Artikel nicht in Rechte Dritter eingreift, inklusive des Copyrights und des Urheberrechtes.
Es ist Sache des Autors, die Nachdruckerlaubnis für Abbildungen, Tabellen usw. aus anderen Publikationen zu beschaffen.
Mit der Annahme des Manuskripts zur Publikation gehen alle Nutzungsrechte auf den Verlag über. Der Verlag hat das Recht, den Artikel in der vorliegenden oder in überarbeiteter Form zu reproduzieren und sich als Erstherausgeber zu bezeichnen. Die Nutzungsrechte sind weltweite Rechte und zeitlich unbegrenzt. Sie beziehen sich sowohl auf alle Print- als auch auf elektronische Offline- und Onlinemedien unter Einschluss des Internets und von Datenbanken/Datenträgern aller Art. Ohne schriftliche Genehmigung des Verlages dürfen diese Publikationen oder Teile daraus nicht in andere Sprachen übersetzt oder in irgendeiner Form mit mechanischen oder elektronischen Mitteln (einschließlich Fotokopie, Tonaufnahme und Mikrofilm) reproduziert oder auf Datenträger oder einem Computersystem gespeichert werden.
Typographische Gestaltung und redaktionelle Bearbeitung werden vom Verlag durchgeführt.

Conflicts of Interest
Die Autoren müssen alle Formen der Unterstützung ihrer Arbeit, inklusive der durch Pharmaunternehmen, angeben; alle Koautoren sollen etwaige Interessenkonflikte offenlegen. Diese Information wird am Ende des Artikels veröffentlicht.

Ethische und rechtliche Voraussetzungen
Manuskripte, bei denen Untersuchungen an Probanden oder Patienten durchgeführt wurden, müssen die Erklärung enthalten, dass das Versuchsprotokoll von einer Ethikkommission genehmigt wurde und den ethischen Standards der Deklaration von Helsinki in ihrer erweiterten Form von 1975 und ihren Zusätzen von 1983, 1989 und 1996 [JAMA 1997;277:925-926] entspricht. Zugleich muss im Manuskripttext auf die Einwilligung der Versuchsperson nach Aufklärung hingewiesen werden. Angaben, die auf die Identität der Person schließen lassen, sind unzulässig.
Im Fall von Tierexperimenten muss von den Autoren angegeben werden, dass diese den jeweils gültigen rechtlichen Standards entsprechen.

Plagiatsrichtlinien
Ob absichtlich oder unabsichtlich, der Diebstahl geistigen Eigentums ist ein ernstes Vergehen. Wir definieren einen Artikel, der zu mindestens 25% mit einer anderen Veröffentlichung übereinstimmt, ohne sie zu zitieren, als Plagiat.
Falls Hinweise auf ein solches Vorgehen vor oder nach der Annahme eines Manuskriptes vorliegen, wird der Autor die Gelegenheit bekommen, dazu Stellung zu nehmen. Wenn seine Argumente nicht zufriedenstellend sind, wird das Manuskript zurückgezogen und dem Autor wird es untersagt, für einen von den zuständigen Editors zu bestimmenden Zeitraum weitere Artikel zu publizieren.

Gliederung
Titelseite: Die Titelseite muss den Titel und Kurztitel der Arbeit in Deutsch und Englisch enthalten.

Autorennamen und -adressen: Die vollständigen Autorennamen mit der jeweiligen Institutsangabe der Autoren, die vollständige Postadresse des Korrespondenzautors sowie die E-Mail-Adresse sollen angegeben sein.

Schlüsselwörter: Zu einer Arbeit gehören 3–5 Schlüsselwörter (Deutsch und Englisch), die möglichst der «Medical Subjects Heading List» des Index Medicus entnommen sein sollen (die Liste ist unter www.nlm.nih.gov erhältlich).

Zusammenfassung: Jedes Manuskript muss eine deutsche und englische Zusammenfassung enthalten, die jeweils 200 Wörter nicht überschreiten. Zusammenfassungen von Originalarbeiten und Übersichtsarbeiten sind zu strukturieren in Hintergrund, Patienten und Methoden (oder Material und Methoden), Ergebnisse und Schlussfolgerungen, die von Kasuistiken in Hintergrund, Fallbericht und Schlussfolgerungen.

Fußnoten: Fußnoten sollten nur in Tabellen verwendet werden.

Geschützte Produkt- bzw. Markennamen: Bei ihrem ersten Auftreten im Text müssen geschützte Produkt- und Markennamen mit einem hochgestellten ® bzw. ™ bezeichnet werden. Die Verantwortung für die korrekte Befolgung dieser Vorschrift liegt ausschließlich beim Autor.

Abbildungen und Tabellen: Tabellen sind Teil des Textes und sollen am Ende des Manuskriptes eingefügt werden. Abbildungen sollen als separate Dateien eingereicht werden. Die Anzahl der Abbildungen und Tabellen sollte limitiert sein, sie sollen den Text illustrieren. Hinweise auf Abbildungen und Tabellen erfolgen im Text mit (Abb. 1) bzw. (Tab. 1). Im Text genannte Informationen bedürfen keiner Wiederholung in einer Tabelle.

Halbtonabbildungen (schwarz-weiß oder farbig) müssen in der endgültigen Größe eine Auflösung von 300 dpi haben, Strichzeichnungen 800–1200 dpi.

Farbabbildungen sind möglich, dem Autor wird jedoch ein Reproduktions- und Druckkostenanteil von EUR 300,– + MWSt. pro Abbildung in Rechnung gestellt.

Referenzen
Das Literaturverzeichnis soll nur die im Text zitierten Publikationen enthalten. Bei Übersichtsarbeiten sollten nicht mehr als 60 Literaturstellen angeben werden.
Die Literatur ist entsprechend der Reihenfolge des Auftretens im Text zu nummerieren. Die Referenzen werden als Zahlen in eckigen Klammern in den Text eingefügt. Bitte nach Möglichkeit alle Autoren einer Arbeit angeben.
Zitiert werden sollen nur Arbeiten, die entweder publiziert oder zur Publikation angenommen sind. Der Passus «in Vorbereitung» oder «persönliche Mitteilung» ist zu vermeiden.
Die Autoren sind für eine korrekte und vollständige Zitierung der Referenzen verantwortlich.
Die Abkürzung der Zeitschriftentitel erfolgt nach dem Index-Medicus-System (www.nlm.nih.gov).
Beispiele zur Abfassung von Literaturzitaten sind zu finden unter www.karger.com/vim_guidelines.

Kosten
Für Artikel, die die maximal vorgesehene Seitenzahl nicht überschreiten, werden keine Druckkosten erhoben (siehe Rubriken und Umfang). Jede weitere angefangene Druckseite wird dem Autor mit EUR 400,– + MWSt. pro Druckseite in Rechnung gestellt.

Druckfahnen
Falls nicht anders vereinbart, werden die Druckfahnen dem Korrespondenzautor zugeschickt und sollen schnellstmöglich zurückgesandt werden. Änderungen in den Druckfahnen, die über die Korrektur von Satzfehlern hinausgehen, werden dem Autor in Rechnung gestellt.

Sonderdrucke
Ein Formular und die Preisliste zur Sonderdruckbestellung werden mit den Druckfahnen versandt. Bestellungen, die nach Drucklegung bei uns eingehen, können nur zu wesentlich höheren Preisen ausgeführt werden.

KARGER
Fax +49 761 4 52 07 14
Information@Karger.com
www.karger.com

Verfügbar unter:
www.karger.com/vim_guidelines